University of Liverpool

Withdrawn from stock

LIVING WITH DEMENTIA:

Living with Dementia

COMMUNITY CARE OF THE ELDERLY MENTALLY INFIRM

C.J. GILLEARD

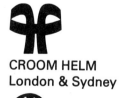

CROOM HELM
London & Sydney

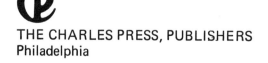

THE CHARLES PRESS, PUBLISHERS
Philadelphia

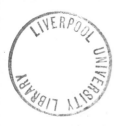

Croom Helm Ltd, Provident House, Burrell Row,
Beckenham, Kent BR3 1AT
Croom Helm Australia Pty Ltd, First Floor,
139 King Street, Sydney, NSW 2001, Australia

British Library Cataloguing in Publication Data

Gilleard, C.J.
   Living with dementia.
   1. Senile dementia—Great Britain
   I. Title
   362.1'989768983'00941   RC524

   ISBN 0–7099–1172–6
   ISBN 0–7099–1173–4 Pbk

and
The Charles Press, Publishers, Suite 14K,
1420 Locust Street, Philadelphia,
Pennsylvania 19102

Library of Congress Catalog Card Number: 84-71615

ISBN 0-914783-05-X Hbk
ISBN 0-914783-07-6 Pbk

Printed and bound in Great Britain

CONTENTS

TO BE READ.

TABLES

ACKNOWLEDGEMENTS

The Scottish Home and Health Department, Chief Scientist's Office, provided a two-year grant to fund the author's surveys of elderly mentally infirm patients and their supporters, and the helpful assistance provided by that body is gratefully acknowledged.

Appreciation of the work conducted by my research colleagues, Janice Whittick, Ken Gledhill and my wife, Esen Gilleard, is made here, not only for the work done, but for many helpful discussions of the issues raised by community care. The related work conducted by Dr John Eagles and Dr Helen Belford has been of great value, and I am glad to acknowledge their contribution to the research project and related issues. Inevitably, the preparation of the manuscript has involved revisions, alterations and additions which have produced a considerable imposition on the time and energy of Mrs Marjory Dodd, whose typing and secretarial assistance is and has been very much appreciated. Finally, additional thanks to Esen, my wife, for her support and help in planning and writing this book.

INTRODUCTION

This book is concerned with the social pressures arising from and current societal responses to the problem of dementia sufferers living in non-institutional settings. The problem is one which has grown more prominent in recent decades as a result of demographic changes in the size and structure of the elderly population. The existence of a constant proportion of institutional places to serve members of the population aged 65 years or over will inevitably lead to an increasing proportion of severely impaired elderly people who remain in the community. This creates a general pressure on families and neighbours to care for such infirm people. However, other social changes are also taking place which may effectively reduce the availability of family support systems. The reduction in the size of families, increased entry into the labour market of women, and the increase in divorce and single-parent families all serve to reduce the availability of the traditional caregiver, the adult woman.

Attempts to provide increasing formal community support – provision of home nursing services, home helps, meals-on-wheels and day centres – is one response to the challenge. Such formal support systems tend to identify need as dependency in instrumental and self-care activities (shopping, cooking, bathing, dressing, etc.). It is here that the problems of dementia fit uneasily into the existing frameworks of support. For dementia is not simply a problem of what the older person can no longer do; it is equally a problem of what such individuals may, or indeed do do. Acts of commission (wandering, abusiveness, urinating inappropriately and so on) rather than acts of omission (inability to dress, wash, feed, walk, etc.) are very often the more significant problems, and it is doubtful whether the models of community services developed for the dependent elderly can meet adequately these sorts of needs.

It is therefore all the more important to identify just what problems do arise in the day-to-day caring of an elderly dementing relative, to gain understanding of the nature of dementia, and how it alters and transforms adult relationships. This requires both adequate clinical description and evaluation and adequate personal records and histories from those living with the dementia sufferer.

My main premiss is that dementia reflects the deterioration and decay of the person or self. Just as personhood or selfhood arises from the organism's interaction with its environment, so selfhood is lost not solely as a decay from within, but also as a decay from without. This does not mean that social and personal relationships cause the decay, but rather that the experience of dementia is one which cannot be separated from the deterioration in personal relationships. The problems of dementia cannot be analysed simply by ever-finer neuropathological investigations of the brain: they exist within the past and present connections that sustain a person, and inevitably vary as much as these relationships do, until the decay from within develops to a point when reduced responsivity to the environment signals the fading of self, and a sad uniformity in the final stages appears.

This, then, is the intention of the book: to cover the interior and exterior processes of dementia, and to set them within the context where they most frequently arise – the community. I have gone on to speculate in the final chapter on what responses can be made to the tragic circumstances that face all those living with dementia.

1 DEMENTIA: ITS INITIAL APPEARANCE

This is how one husband described the onset of his wife's dementia:

> I didn't really notice, until much later, but looking back, now, I can find things that happened . . . she used to be a good card player, you see, especially at solo whist, she belonged to a club, went every week, twice a week, and several times she was forgetting the numbers of the cards, and – she had a pretty good memory for that, for knowing which cards are out – and eventually she could only remember the face cards – looking back it was the beginning, in fact, and that was so many years ago – ten years anyway – but eventually she had to leave, then she gravitated to bingo, but even that was getting too much for her – but we didn't think no more of that, either, for some reason, but eventually it just gradually came, she would just stand in the kitchen, and wonder why she was there, she was going to do something and just didn't remember what she was there for – this was the time I began to get anxious about her – she could still do things but she forgot very often where she was and what she was going to do . . . and since then it's just been a gradual process . . .
>
> She could still carry out certain tasks, she could still wash herself and things like that, but she wasn't so able, at that particular time, then her sister came to live with us and she did the cooking, so she didn't need to do anything, for about a year, till her sister left, and I had to take it over then – and I was still doing a part-time job at that time, for hours in the afternoon, but she was always very anxious, she used to go outside, and she wasn't too good on her feet then, shaky for some reason, she always visited the neighbours, always went to the neighbours' homes, and they said it was all right, but you felt it was getting, you know, a bit of an annoyance to them – as soon as I left, as soon as, the neighbour said, as soon as you're away – she was out of the door, and I felt it was getting a bit too much, relying on neighbours all the time, and so I eventually left my work to look after her properly . . .
>
> Now she can't do a thing, now I've got to get her out of bed,

and wash her, and dress her, every morning, and take all her wet things off every morning, it's a wet bed, but as I say the whole thing has come on so gradually over the years . . . and well at the moment, you see, it's all right, during the day, mostly, except it's a one-sided affair, really . . .

This picture of a gradual loss of competence, from the relatively complex skills of solo whist playing to the loss of basic dressing and toiletting habits, represents one important dimension in the development of dementia. But it is not by any means the only one, nor invariably the first one recognised by the family. This is how one woman described the early changes she noticed in her husband:

Well, he started on the motorists, what business had they parking in front of the door, and telling them to take their cars away or he would get the police. He would use very bad language . . . it would be about beginning at that time, you see, and with the children, too, that came – we have a little garden and of course if the children came near the garden, he would tell them to clear out and things like that, and threaten them – once a ball came into the garden and instead of handing it back, he pitched it right across the road . . . and not so long ago, he threw a hoe at one of the children in the street, and then I had a neighbour at the other end of the street and she came along and said he had threatened their son, and when she spoke to him he threatened her . . . but however, since then she's recognised that he's not just normal . . . anyway, in fact, I said to him, I'll have no friends left in the street if you carry on like this . . . well, for a long time he'd always had a bad memory for names, for people, he would come in and he would say to me, 'I saw, e', and then he would stop and he wouldn't remember who it was. I had to guess who it was, and because I couldn't, he would get himself into a rage . . . and other things, he never did much shopping at all, except for his papers, and he'd get me two pints of milk, well sometimes he would come back with four, you know, with two cartons instead of one, and just recently he said, well, he would get the milk, but where's the flagon?

For this wife, the change in character, the bad temper and impulsive reactions were odd and upsetting; it was the appearance of 'new' behaviour that indicated all was not well, rather than the disappearance of existing skills. Even the lapses of memory were subordinated to the emotional distress occasioned by them.

It is probably the case that almost all family carers will identify the onset of dementia with either the loss of existing skills or knowledge or the occurrence of odd or disturbed behaviour. For children not living with their parent, it may be a distressed call to say that people have got into their house, or on visiting their parent to hear him or her express strange ideas about neighbours, or even a bizarre account of animals, clowns or noises seen or heard in the bedroom the previous night.

As an example of the slow occurrence of oddness, this account was given by a daughter of the early stages of her mother's dementia. After a burglary at the daughter's house, her mother, who was living on her own, started telling her about 'odd people who were up to no good'. Stories like this became more frequent – on the train she had seen a man dressed as a woman; the man across the road was doing jobs at night; and so on. Later, she burned several documents relating to her house, saying that she did not like looking at them. This was followed by questions about her money – what had she (the daughter) done with her money? This developed into persecutory ideas. The daughter and a neighbour of the mother's were stealing her money, they were in league, locking her into the house with a Chubb bolt, from the inside. Everything in the house was now locked, and the mother kept everything about her person, stuffed in her handbag or pinned to her cardigan. People were having picnics in her house, people were wearing her clothes, people were coming into the house while she was asleep. Throughout this time, the mother lived independently, travelled on public transport, visited her daughter and generally coped with self-care and the necessary acts of daily life without any obvious cognitive failure. The mother insisted there was nothing wrong with her, she was all right in the head, and knew what they (daughter, family and neighbours) were up to.

Later, memory lapses became apparent, but even then the embarrassing persecutory accusations remained to the fore, until accidents in the home due to forgetfulness took over, and embarrassment and distress were replaced by the daughter's mounting anxieties about her mother's safety.

For those living with the patient, it is more often the lapses in memory, or mistakes made, which occur with increasing severity and lead to a growing concern. One woman was surprised to find her husband, returning from a short holiday, ask if there was any letter from his mother, who had died years before.

In retrospect, events such as a holiday or illness or accident become the starting-point of the dementia, though often there will have been signs much earlier of a gradual loss of mental competence and increasing absent-mindedness. At the time, such changes are frequently passed off as due to ageing, and it is only the sudden abnormality which causes alarm. In other cases, the mental impairment arises sharply and concretely, when the patient has a stroke, and fails to regain normal mental functions. Though the event is sudden, it often causes less anxiety because there is likely to be an immediate understanding of the changes and how they have been brought about.

Gilhooley (1980) has pointed out the frequent confusion most supporting relatives have over causation. She found that most of the relatives she interviewed associated the start of dementia with a physical illness, operation or some particular emotional event. She describes how several caregivers talked about the dementia in terms of morality; 'they could not understand how or why this had happened as the patient had always been a good person'. She also points out the hazy chronology that may exist in describing causality, mentioning a caregiver who 'tied the start of the disorder to a house-breaking incident . . . which . . . had occurred several years before there were signs of loss of memory or disorientation'.

In one of our own studies (Gilleard and Watt, 1982) we found that half of the caregiving relatives had no idea of what caused their dependant's dementia; most of the reasons given were either 'old age' or 'hardening of the arteries'. This latter explanation was also the most frequently given by Gilhooley's sample of caregivers.

The problems of accurately dating and describing the onset of dementia are important for both clinical and research reasons. Clinically, the issue is one of early identification. Over 20 years ago, Williamson *et al.* (1964) showed that more than half of all the cases of dementia in their survey were unknown to the general practitioners. What may be the problem is both a lack of awareness on the part of the elderly patient, and a lack of understanding and recognition on the part of the relatives visiting or living with the dementing person. At what point is it reasonable to expect relatives to distinguish between the 'normal' lapses of memory and grasp in old age, and the more malignant impairments of dementia? Indeed, is it clear that such a distinction really exists? Bergmann *et al.* (1971)

have shown that over one-third of suspected dementia patients in the community (suspected, that is, by clinicians) remained three years later, perfectly competent, while a further third remained still 'under suspicion'. Time does not always reveal the answer. Our own studies – to be described later in the book – indicate that it is often the case that a gap of over two or three years may occur between the relative suspecting all is not well, and their contacting a doctor about the problem. This problem may of course be compounded by denial of the problems and their implications. Barnes *et al.* (1981) described one wife of a dementing person as saying: 'For the first year I completely denied the whole thing. I tried to explain the changes in my husband as being due to poor eyesight caused by glaucoma. My friends supported me and kept reassuring me that there couldn't be anything wrong with him.'

Although many clinicians remain hopeful of using new or existing drug remedies which might prove successful if only cases could be identified in the 'early stages', it is true to say that those early stages are very often difficult to pin down, even for the person living close at hand. This raises a problem for research, of course. Establishing the 'age of onset' is considered important (a) to determine the likely course of a dementia, (b) to examine the significance of differing ages of onset on both the course and outcome of this condition, and (c) to understand the effectiveness of therapeutic intervention carried out at early stages.

Criteria laid down by researchers regarding the determination of onset are often vague, and inevitably rely upon relatives' recall of changes which, as may be seen, are subject to what Gilhooley (1980) calls an 'effort after meaning' on the part of the relatives. Thus Semple, Smith and Swash (1982), reporting the results of interviews with relatives of early dementia patients found 'some relatives were hesitant about stating when symptoms appeared', presumably because of their own uncertainties. These authors compared relatives' and doctors' reports of illness duration, and found agreement within three months occurred only twice in their sample of 14, while half had levels of disagreement by two years or more. Clearly, retrospective reports are not very reliable means of dating onset. It is difficult to prescribe any set criterion for determining what constitutes the onset of dementia. LaRue and Jarvik (1980) have shown, for example, differences in cognitive performance occurring 20 years before the diagnosis of dementia was made. Suggestions of an early cognitive impairment considerably pre-dating clinical symptoms have also been made in the case of Huntington's chorea, usually considered as a type of pre-senile dementia. Reisberg and his colleagues (1982) have suggested a 'very mild cognitive decline' stage as representing the onset of dementia – determined by subjective complaints of poor memory, and objective psychometric deficits – but it is questionable whether the subjective complaints of poor memory are typical for late-life dementias. Abrams has shown that for the over-75s the majority will complain of forgetfulness and poor memory (Abrams, 1978). This simply serves to emphasise an important difference between the unusual occurrence of dementia in middle age and the less distinctive development of dementia in late life. It is not only ageing expectations that highlight dementia in mid-life and mask it in later life. An additional factor seems also to be the question of insight, which is often less apparent in late-life dementias. The extent to which the loss or retention of insight is related to the existence of differential patterns of neuropathology is still open to doubt. One alternative model is that personal adjustment strategies also intervene – contrasting the paranoid response of 'where did you put my keys?' to the depressive 'oh dear, I've lost my keys, I'm so forgetful', but again one may postulate that the former reflects a more complex cognitive loss than the latter – failing to remember, and failing to recognise the memory failure, while the latter is the more restricted incompetence of failing to remember.

In our study of 129 new referrals for psychogeriatric day care, we recorded the relative frequency with which various types of signs and symptoms were recalled by relatives as indicating the onset of dementia. In over half the cases (52 per cent) cognitive loss was observed, closely followed by signs of physical ill-health (46 per cent), with changes in social behaviour (24 per cent) and psychopathology (29 per cent) described in about one-quarter of the cases. None of these is naturally exclusive, but it is interesting to note the high frequency with which signs of physical ill-health were observed at the outset by the supporters. One example is the husband who, when asked how the dementia began, said 'Well, what happened, she was very, very white, very white and getting thin, and by the look of her I thought it was bloodlessness . . .' Others would mention falls or unsteadiness, or fatigue. In general, spouses and siblings tended to identify cognitive loss and physical ill-health as the more frequent signs of onset, whereas adult children and nieces tended to report changes in social behaviour (household neglect, embarrassing displays of temper or hostility) and psychopathology (hallucinations, delusions, depression) relatively more frequently, and physical ill-health less so than the elderly caregivers. Whether this reflects a differing perspective, differing concerns and differing levels of tolerance is an open question. It may well be that the presence of a spouse simply reduces the frequency of psychopathological manifestations in the elderly person at the early stages of their dementia, because the insecurity is less in such households.

It is tempting to reduce the heterogeneity of the presentation of dementia into typologies and to seek endogenous neuropathological factors as accounting for the differing forms. Yet it may be more likely that historical and environmental factors account for much more of the variabilities and uncertainties surrounding the recognition that 'something is wrong' in the early stages, and that only as dementia progresses does the underlying pathology determine a homogeneous pathway of ultimate decline.

Wells (1978) states: 'dementia remains a clinical syndrome that must be established by clinical evaluation'. This chapter will duly focus on the clinical manifestations of dementia, and is based on the author's assumption that the development of understanding concerning the cognitive, emotional and behavioural deficits that make up dementia is not dependent upon any precise delimitation of the origins and nature of the underlying cerebral pathology. It is important nevertheless to recognise that the clinical syndrome of dementia may be associated with a variety of presumptive organic pathologies, and that, although primary cerebral atrophy remains the single most likely source of neuropathological deficit, many other aetiologies exist. Table 2.1 presents, in summary form, the results of aetiological investigation in 464 cases of presumed dementia, from five studies carried out in the last decade, together with the results of one large-scale investigation of possible dementia patients referred for brain scans using computerised tomography.

It should be noted that a 'neurological bias' to referrals and the existence of a substantial number of under-70s are likely to lead to the over-representation of rare, reversible and drink-related pathologies. Smith and Kiloh (1981) reported 90 per cent of their patients aged over 65 to have a presumed primary atrophic dementia, while Bradshaw, Thomson and Campbell (1983) found less than 8 per cent of their patients aged 75 and over with suspected dementias had potentially treatable lesions, and 5 per cent of this age-group had a 'normal scan'. A discussion of possible aetiologies for the primary atrophy (nowadays going under the banner of 'dementia of the Alzheimer type', or DAT) can be found in recent articles by Schneck, Reisberg and Ferris (1982) and Rossor (1982).

Wells has recently advocated that a greater interest should be shown in all three aspects of change occurring in dementia – the behavioural, affective and cognitive elements – rather than, as at present, most interest being directed to the purely cognitive area (Wells, 1982). One may go further, and agree with Symonds, that dementia is not simply the loss of some particular function, but is in essence the loss of the person (Symonds, 1981). Using the term 'global' to describe the deterioration taking place as people dement

Table 2.1: Results from the Clinical Investigation of 464 Cases of Suspected Dementia and Computerised Tomographic (CT) Findings from a Further Sample of 500 Suspected Dementia Cases

Presumed condition	n	(%)	CT study	Na	(%)
Atrophic primary dementia	220	(47.5)	Atrophy	180	(36.0)
Cerebral arteriopathic dementia	44	(9.5)	Multiple infarcts	129	(25.0)
Alcohol-related dementia	44	(9.5)	Recent infarct	19	(4.0)
Korsakoff's syndrome	11	(2.0)	Alcohol abuse	31	(6.0)
Dementia: uncertain	14	(3.0)			
Hydrocephalic dementia	23	(5.0)	Hydrocephalus	6	(1.0)
Intracranial mass/tumour	19	(4.0)	Intracranial mass/tumour	42	(8.5)
Huntingdon's chorea	15	(3.0)	Huntington's chorea	3	(<1.0)
Parkinson's disease	4	(1.0)	Parkinson's disease	19	(4.0)
Jakob-Creutzfeldt dementia	3	(<1.0)			
Intracranial haemorrhage	3	(<1.0)	Intracranial haemorrhage		(<1.0)
Post-traumatic dementia	8	(2.0)			
Post-encephalitic dementia	3	(<1.0)			
Drug toxicity	8	(2.0)			
Thyroid disease	5	(1.0)			
Other systemic diseases	2	(<1.0)			
Other neurological disorders	8	(2.0)			
Pseudo-dementia (affective illness)	21	(4.5)			
Pseudo-dementia (psychosis)	9	(2.0)	'Normal'	80	(16.0)

Notes: N^a exceeds 500 due to some patients with 'multiple signs'.

Sources: Results from clinical investigation of 464 cases of suspected dementia from Victoratos, Lenman and Herzberg (1977), Wells (1978) and Smith and Kiloh (1981). Results from computerised tomographic findings of suspected dementia cases from Bradshaw, Thomson and Campbell (1983).

both recognises yet somehow hides this fact.

The study of the syndrome of dementia requires consideration of what constitutes the self, what makes a person, what holds together the acts of an individual to give him or her personal integrity, consistency and ultimately value. Guntrip (1971) speaks of the importance of personal relatedness, and the growth of self as the growth of personal reality within oneself, a point echoed in Foulds concept of personhood (Foulds, 1976). This sense of personal reality seems to be the essence of what decays as dementia progresses. This personal reality seems to depend upon the intactness of memory, the ability to continue to interpret the present within the structure of personal experience in the past, and the ability to extend this continuity to one's future intentions. The confusion that surrounds the dementing person is a confusion over reference points, both current and historical, which dislocates actions, misperceives experience and loses the thread that gives meaning and intentionality to behaviour, which taken globally reflects a fundamental loss of relatedness, to both the physical and social environment.

This loss is not simply one of memory, in the sense of an inability to learn or to store information. Patients who, as a result of brain trauma, lose the ability to update their knowledge, who fail to learn and store anything new, are not demented, nor do they appear demented. One may argue that their self does not, or cannot develop, yet it is retained.

Equally, patients who, as a result of head injury, become increasingly self-centred, immature and shallow, are not perceived to be, or to have demented. Their behaviour may be impulsive, abstract codes of conduct may be easily overruled by the inability to delay gratification, yet however much personality change is recorded, the remaining person retains a self and a grasp on reality and continues to develop.

Finally, mentally handicapped people, whose language is limited to a few stereotyped utterances, who struggle to put on a coat, and who precariously learn to carry a plate from the table, held high and awkwardly as if it would slip at any moment, nevertheless do not seem demented. They recognise their place in the family, the familiar route home, they seek a limited but meaningful relation with people around them.

Yet in some way the static deficits observable in the amnesic person, the disinhibited brain-damaged person and the intellectually handicapped person all share similarities with the pattern of dynamic impairments observable in the dementing person. It is the onslaught from all sides that seems to take away any opportunity to maintain some form of orientation and personal integrity.

Cognitive Changes

The memory failure, particularly the failure to remember what one has done, is a prominent feature of dementia. Miller's work on memory in Alzheimer's disease clearly suggests a failure of new information to reach any permanent storage, despite being initially apprehended (Miller, 1971). But forgetfulness in dementia is unlikely to be simply a 'storage' problem, and further work by Miller and others employing cueing at recall (e.g. saying the first letter of a word to be recalled) suggested that a retrieval deficit is also present which may be as important as the difficulties in retaining new information (Miller, 1975; Diesfeldt, 1978; Morris, Wheatley and Britton, 1983). The existence of a retrieval deficit seems in any case necessary to account for the dementing person's growing failure to recall events from the past which clearly had been adequately stored in the first place.

Such problems over retrieval may, in turn, lead to additional difficulty in correctly labelling new information: the forgetting that one is on holiday makes the interpretation of waking up in new surroundings harder to assimilate, and enhances its novelty effects, providing additional anxiety-arousing properties for such disoriented experiences. Experimental studies also point to the difficulty for dementing persons in acquiring information as a result of inadequacies in accessing existing knowledge structures that would facilitate encoding processes (Weingartner *et al.*, 1981).

Such a failure to place experience, to relate the here and now with the recent and remote past, does in itself make new learning harder, if not impossible, besides providing the basis for misinterpretation and 'disinhibition of recall' (i.e. the failure to recognise 'false' recall). Memory failures represent, therefore, negative errors – failure to recall someone's name, or what one has just said or done – as well as positive errors, which may be expressed in the belief that one's mother is still alive, that the hospital is a school playground, that the doctor or nurse is a well-loved friend. The inability to learn, to grasp new information, is compounded by a more malignant inability to recall and use past information and knowledge to maintain the quality of relatedness that one may define as maintaining selfhood.

A further clinical feature of the memory impairment in dementia is the problem of forgetting what one is doing. While the failure of relating present to past experience, and vice versa, has been discussed, the failure to relate present behaviour to future intended actions is frequently observed in dementia, and, from time to time, in all of us. In part, this is a failure to remember what one has done, as well as a failure to remember the goal or purpose to which past and present behaviour was intended. Most commonly, it appears that an intention or purpose is formed, which has initiated the beginnings of the behavioural sequence, but with the failure to maintain or recall the overall purposes or goal, current behaviour loses the internal reference points of where to proceed next, leaving the individual stranded in the middle of a piece of behaviour whose links are broken. The dementing person pauses in the kitchen, bemused and lost, unable to generate any continuity for his or her actions. At this point, the result may be the simple cessation of action, or the production of new, unrelated behavioural acts, cued by some external feature of the environment.

Such failures reflect a forgetting of internally produced plans, purposes or intentions, which have been formed, but have either faded or become disrupted by new events after those produced by the very actions set off by the purpose or plan in the first place. Having walked into the kitchen with the purpose of washing up, the dementing person's experience of entering the kitchen seems almost to weaken their ability to access the original plan. Such forgetfulness of plans and intentions is rarely observed in other chronic amnesic disorders, such as Korsakoff's psychosis, and yet in many ways it produces the discontinuity, distractability and lack of purposiveness that most distinguishes individuals with dementia from those with more localised cognitive disabilities. It is also harder to examine and test for, since it is forgetfulness not of externally generated information (dates, names, where objects have been placed, etc.) nor even of one's own actions, but the information which is forgotten is internally generated and the nature of that information is not easily determined nor is it accessible to experimental manipulation. One may well envisage that such memory failures are both more severe than the usual amnesia for events, and involve perhaps different mechanisms for their origins.

How far other cognitive changes represent separate dysfunction is uncertain. Several workers have pointed to the presence of so-called 'focal' deficits in dementia (Lauter and Meyer, 1968; McDonald, 1969; Constantinidis, 1978). These reflect disturbances in expressive speech and writing and impairment of spatial and bodily orientation. The former is illustrated by one dementing lady who would go into a shop and ask for 'a yellow pac-a-mac', or 'a packet of the Moppet Show'. Not only was her speech affected but her writing skills were much deteriorated, though in other ways she did not seem grossly confused. The loss of bodily orientation is also demonstrated by some dementing people's inability to recognise their own image in the mirror, or to relate the legs or sleeves of an article of clothing to their own arms or legs, resulting in confused attempts to get dressed.

The similarity of these accentuated deficits in symbolic expression and positional orientation to the effects of discrete lesions in the cerebral cortex has raised questions regarding their significance to the pattern of developing neuropathology underlying dementia. There is reason to believe that the disruption of such overlearned skills as speech, dressing and writing reflects a poorer prognosis and more rapid course to the deterioration (Kasniak *et al.*, 1978; Naguib and Levy, 1982).

Considering the loss of general intellectual functioning, numerous studies of dementing people's performance on standardised tests of intelligence attest to a marked reduction in intellectual performance (Miller, 1977). Typical also is the finding that measures of abstract conceptual reasoning and novel problem-solving are more affected than those relying upon acquired mental skills, and the retrieval of old knowledge (Inglis, 1958). Such evidence points to a failure to develop new knowledge and new problem-solving strategies, in contrast to a preserved ability to apply existing knowledge and strategies. This is probably consistent with work on memory impairment, where the learning deficit (a failure to update one's intelligence) precedes the retrieval deficit (a failure to apply one's intelligence). Equally, it is harder to learn information to solve problems of less personal relevance, rather than those of more personal meaning. The frequent loss of abstract interests – in politics, current affairs, theatre, TV, etc. – is often commented upon by relatives, as though the self first loses its relatedness to a more distant, impersonal and conceptually more abstract environment, before ultimately failing to maintain personal concrete knowledge and interests, with disinterest in friends and family eventually leading to disinterest in oneself and one's physical self-maintenance.

Such changes reinforce the view that the underlying cognitive changes in learning, thinking and remembering provide the basis for much of the overt behavioural changes observed by the caregivers of dementing people. It seems likely, however, that the occurrence of retrieval failures and the inability to follow what one once found easy to grasp has an emotional impact which may be likened to 'learned helplessness' (Seligman, 1975). The frustration of cognitive intentions due to one's own cognitive inefficiency is a cause of frequent distress, rage and irrational accusations, which contribute to a picture of emotional and motivational abnormalities, which, as Wells (1982) points out, have not been fully investigated. This frustration may, in turn, lead to the reduced use of goal-planning, because of the failure of such plans to be reinforced by successful execution; this results in what some workers have termed 'cognitive abulia'.

Emotional Changes

Although there have not been extensive studies of mood and motivational changes in dementia, several psychiatrists have examined the type of mood changes occurring in dementia. Liston (1977) observed that amongst a series of patients who eventually received a diagnosis of pre-senile dementia, more than half presented with significant affective (emotional) disturbance in their early psychiatric contacts. One-third of his sample had received an original diagnosis of an affective disorder (depression or anxiety) and had received treatment for this. Reifler, Larson and Hanley (1982) screened a series of geriatric psychiatry outpatients and found that although over 80 per cent were mentally impaired (presumably dementing), 26 per cent demonstrated sufficient symptoms of emotional upset that they could be classified as having an affective disorder (depressive illness). Interestingly, with progressively severe cognitive impairment, the prevalence of depressive illness declined – 33 per cent of the mildly impaired being considered to have a depressive illness, 23 per cent of the moderately impaired and only 12 per cent of the severely impaired.

Extreme anxiety and agitation are also reported to occur, often in the form of a catastrophic reaction to some failure of competence, and a general sense of worry and apprehension over the shifting pattern of impairment that some people recognise occurring in the early stages. It is difficult to know how common sustained emotional distress is, especially in the elderly person with a gradually progressive failure of mental competence.

The personal suffering of the dementing person may be over-interpreted by the distress caused to the carer by seeing someone they may have loved and respected slowly lose those qualities they once admired them for. An impression gained, though by no means substantiated empirically, is that earlier onset of decline produces greater distress in the person, possibly because such decline occurs more rapidly and is therefore more easily recognised and appreciated by the person. Equally, if there is more evident loss of established skills, with only a gradual reduction in overall mental competence, the deficiency may be more striking and frustrating.

Depression and anxiety are also conspicuously absent in some people, and it is their apparent emotional indifference that is the more striking. The so-called frontal lobe syndrome – associating motivational deficiencies of apathy, lack of initiation and purpose, and emotional shallowness with atrophy of the frontal lobe – has been postulated as a reason for the enhanced vulnerability of the dementing person living alone to come to medical attention earlier (Blumenthal, 1979). She suggests that such deficiencies in sustaining internal goal-planning more easily lead to self-neglect and excess disabilities, in the absence of a partner or other relative providing a cueing function, for example, prompting the person to get up, to wash, to eat and so forth.

Such motivational deficiencies certainly play an important part in reducing the effectiveness of formal support services. Thus one elderly man would regularly have meals delivered to his house; these would then accumulate, since he felt apparently no motivation to eat them. He did not seem depressed, and when prompted by the warden of the sheltered accommodation unit where he lived, he would quite competently eat his lunches up. His memory at this time was not grossly impaired, but recalling the fact that the meal had been delivered seemed not to prompt him to eat – the cue or directive had to come from outside.

This loss of initiative and internal goal-setting may present as a quite separate impairment from that of memory and intellectual skills, and yet it may prove, as Blumenthal suggests, the principal handicap to an independent life in the community.

Behavioural Changes

While much of the cognitive, emotional and motivational changes may seem to account for the observable behavioural impairments in dementia, certain behavioural problems exist which seem worthy of independent consideration, particularly those of restlessness, wandering, incontinence, and aggressive and abusive behaviour – what Burnside has called 'symptomatic behaviours of the elderly' (Burnside, 1980). One might also add to this list the voracious eating that a minority of dementing people exhibit periodically.

It is apparent from many studies of behavioural ratings made on dementing patients that a dimension of behavioural disturbance emerges as quite independent from the impairment and dependency usually linked to the deterioration of cognitive function (Gilleard, 1984a). It is also the case that, unlike the progressive deterioration in self-care and behavioural competence, such disturbance is by no means a progressive feature. The present author, in a series of longitudinal studies of behaviour change in dementing patients, found that changes in socially disruptive behaviour did not show a pattern of linear increase over time, nor did they fall into a dimension of cumulative development – that is, there was no evidence of a sequential pattern in the type or degree of disturbance (Gilleard, 1978). As Burnside (1980) has pointed out, very little study has been made of these problems and much of what follows relies more on clinical rather than empirically based evidence.

Wandering and Restlessness

In a factor analytic study of the problems reported by supporters of the elderly mentally infirm, Gilleard, Boyd and Watt (1982) found that a separate 'dimension' made up of day-time and night-time wandering emerged, independent of both the dimension of dependency or impaired self-care and that of behavioural disturbance. From this finding, it would appear that wandering is not a behaviour closely linked to either the degree of dementia, or the extent of disruptive and disturbing behaviour. Burnside (1980) has suggested that wandering may often be 'a self-assigned exercise program' amongst the elderly who have always led active lives. One wife of a dementing patient described spending much of her day taking her husband on bus journeys in Edinburgh, as a way of reducing his restless pacing and desire to get out of the house. Another patient, a man in his sixties suffering from Pick's disease (a rare form of pre-senile dementia) would regularly turn up at his old workplace to see ex-colleagues. In this case, because of his well-preserved spatial orientation he would manage these journeys relatively safely. Sometimes he would set off from hospital and arrive back hours later, with no coherent explanation of where he had been, or how he had travelled, though from indirect reports it seemed likely that he had gone some quite considerable distances.

Often, however, the sudden disappearance from home of an elderly mentally infirm person, unsuitably dressed, is the cause for extreme anxiety in the supporter, and results in major restrictions on the person's activity, the supporter not daring to risk a recurrence.

Wandering may occur in at least three separate contexts. First, there is the problem of wandering as restless activity-seeking, more common in men, when a physically fit, but mentally incompetent man cannot sit still, and appears to be continually trying to stay active and on the move. Such individuals may always have been used to a high level of activity and, while not having clear goals of where they are going, seem nevertheless to want to get out or to be on the move. Usually their gait is quite steady and they show no major mobility problems.

A second problem is that of the 'stalker of old haunts'. Again, the person is usually male and has been used to a routine of going out, visiting friends, going to the local club and so forth. The habit of going visiting remains, but the competence of successfully making the visit and return may become increasingly fragile, and such individuals may find themselves getting lost after straying or being distracted from their regular route.

A third type of wandering results from disorientation and an inability to sustain the goals of one's actions. Here, it is often wandering confined to the house, or immediate neighbourhood. The individual may have got up with a reason in mind, then forgotten and become distracted by other stimuli, leading them to potter about looking around the house with no obvious motive, or occasionally, prompted by insecurity, to search for some object, letter or document that becomes almost fixed as an obsession, and which produces anxiety and agitation because the object searched for cannot be found.

Perhaps the element of mobility determines the variable occurrence of wandering in dementing people. Any unsteadiness or fall can produce exaggerated anxiety about walking, which leads to a marked reluctance to venture any distance from a resting place, and essentially confounds any desire to wander off. A second 'restraining' influence is the extreme separation anxiety that some dementing people experience, leading them to seek to maintain close visible contact with their supporter, who acts as a permanent orienting cue to their whereabouts and personal security.

Incontinence

Often distressing to both the mentally infirm person himself, and to his supporter, incontinence is a frequent accompaniment of dementia. Surveys of hospitalised psychogeriatric patients suggest that the prevalence of regular urinary incontinence in the population may be around 40 – 50 per cent (Gilleard, 1981), and episodes of incontinence (once, twice or three times per week) may occur in a further 20 per cent (McLaren *et al.*, 1981). In surveys of dementia supporters, the prevalence of some incontinence seems to be lower (see Chapter 5), averaging around 25 – 35 per cent.

One problem posed by the occurrence of incontinence in dementia is whether it reflects the severity of the dementia, or whether its occurrence is largely independent of the degree of mental deterioration: more specifically, would all cases of dementia eventually become incontinent, providing they survive to reach the severe stages of dementia? It seems likely that the difficulty in answering such problems lies in the occurrence of incontinence relatively early in some people, while in others it represents the end-point of a long slow decline.

Three possible settings are apparent: incontinence arising from a 'localised' physical or psychological abnormality coexisting with dementia, such as infection, prolapse, constipation, severe depression, etc.; incontinence arising from the indirect consequences of other disabilities, especially mobility problems, making reaching the toilet more difficult, dressing problems, making toiletting more difficult, and confusion, making the goal-pursuing element of going to the toilet, orientating oneself to the toilet and so forth, more difficult; and finally, incontinence arising directly from loss of learned bladder control due to cortical atrophy. While the latter may reflect the irremediable deterioration process, it may be that the loss of control due to mental and organic deterioration can be considerably delayed by adequate health-care monitoring and the reduction of obstacles making use of the toilet difficult or frustrating.

Aggression and Hostility

Problems of overt physical aggression and assaultiveness are most often the province of institutional rather than home care. The interaction of confused, disinhibited and disoriented persons in wards and other institutional living areas inevitably creates a setting for sudden acts of aggression and violent outbursts, which rarely occur at home, mostly because disorientation is less, and security is greater. Often, it is not the physically aggressive act that is disconcerting to supporters, but rather the significance of the act – a husband who puts his hands round his wife's neck may cause pain, but the more painful discovery that someone so close, someone so loved and respected, can behave towards their partner as if they were a stranger, an unrecognised intruder, can be much more distressing.

As with the other symptomatic behaviours, aggression and hostility can be viewed as having very different contextual settings. Perhaps the most frequent are disinhibited over-reactions to frustration, when the dementing person gets into a rage because of a name that they cannot remember, or an article of clothing they cannot put on, or because of some unexpected change in routine. The mixture of threat and frustration represented by such overt failures of competence can lead to temper outbursts which are then poorly controlled. The presence of non-intimate strangers or visitors may, however, inhibit such outbursts, due to over-learned social skills, whereas the presence of intimates may reduce the likelihood of such restraining influences.

Next, there is the hostility of extrapunitive accusations – a daughter has stolen her mother's money, people have ganged up to throw someone out of the house, a wife is poisoning her husband's food, etc. Misinterpretations of events can provide external sources of blame for internally caused incompetence producing an 'adaptive paranoia' (Lieberman, 1975), which reduces the distress of fully recognising the extent to which one can no longer control and cope with one's immediate environment. The caring relative may find it especially hard to adjust when such accusations are made to others, or shouted out in public. Since such attempts to cover one's own incompetence and insecurity are frequently early rather than late accompaniments of dementia, the accusations may be more plausibly received by other people as the dementing person's credibility is not yet eroded by obvious cognitive incompetence. Also, in the absence of major cognitive impairment, such behaviour may be seen as more deliberately intended, in the eyes of the supporters. Finally, aggression may emerge as a defensive reaction to threatening intrusions of personal space and independence. Bathing may be resisted, because of the fear of being burned, or drowned. Dressing may be resisted because of the explicit evidence of incompetence, which the elderly person seems to deny or, at least, fails to recognise. 'Why are you trying to dress me, I can manage myself.' Attempts to come in and do housework may equally be verbally and physically repelled, due either to the threat of incompetence or the fear that another's imposition of order may further threaten the elderly person's grasp of and orientation to their surroundings.

Many other unique behavioural problems emerge during the course of some people's dementing process. The use of antipsychotic medication is often proposed as a means of sedating the person, though it offers little in the way of adequately analysing and coming to grips with such behaviour problems. That said, it is probably true that such behaviours are sufficiently stressful that they alienate the carer from their dementing relative, and make it more acceptable for clinicians to offer such treatment, to make life easier for the family. The effectiveness of such management procedures is not clearly established, however, and the side-effects associated with these medications can lead to more serious health problems (Barnes *et al.*, 1982).

The existence of both emotional and behavioural pathology has led to an interest in classifying the psychopatholgoy of dementia, aside from the central cognitive loss and interest, which can be seen as having both beneficial and harmful consequences. It is beneficial to increase clinicians' appreciation of the multiple problems and presentations occurring as the elderly person dements, but it is harmful to move from such descriptive approaches to one of diagnostic classifications, which seem to be consequent upon this style of investigation, as though describing a typology of dementia provides an adequate account of the pathology. The 'heterogeneity of dementia' (cf. McDonald, 1969) may be valuably recognised, but it seems doubtful whether such recognition can be usefully crystal-lised into subtyping of dementia.

Psychopathological Syndromes

Several psychiatric writers have described the existence of different types of dementia, based upon prominent psychopathological features, such as the depressed type, the hypochondriacal type, the simple dementia type and the paranoid type (Muller, 1967; Wertheimer, 1974). Some attempts have been made to examine these typologies using multivariate techniques of analysis, notably factor and cluster analysis (Jonsson, Waldton and Malhammer, 1973; Ballinger, Reid and Heather, 1982). While these studies have identified several independent dimensions or factors of impairment in dementing patients, the clustering of these dimensions of psy-chopathology has yielded little of significance beyond the recog-nition that psychopathology in dementia is multidimensional – a point made at the beginning of this chapter.

It is possible from the latter two empirical studies to argue that paranoid and depressive symptomatology may be limited to a group or groups of dementing patients, in contrast to other dementing patients who remain relatively free of additional psychiatric symp-tomatology, but even so the significance of such symptom patterns remains dubious, for several reasons. In the first place, paranoid or depressive reactions may simply characterise the earlier stages of dementia, when the individual either attempts to rationalise their incompetence or becomes distressed by it, until the dementia pro-gresses beyond the stage where awareness of the mistakes and errors is lost – psychopathology thus representing a stage, rather than a subtype of dementia. Secondly, such features may simply reflect pre-morbid personality traits, which have become exag-gerated by the dementing process – a point recognised by Ballinger *et al.* (1982) in their study. Thirdly, it may reflect little more than the professional habit of labelling patients in line with one's own parti-cular discipline, in the same way that some nurses will label patients as 'wanderers' or 'moaners' or 'soilers'. The selective attention to certain features in the behaviour of such patients may thus under-play other factors, and involve a reinterpretation of behaviours in line with other psychiatric patients. The release of psychopathology in dementia may simply be as varied as the development of psychiatric syndromes in the pre-dementing population.

Gustafson and Hagberg (1975) studied a group of patients with pre-senile dementia and examined the relationship between various factors of cognitive impairment and functional psychopathology. They observed considerable highly significant intercorrelations between their 14 factors; for example, the depression factor was negatively correlated with both cognitive impairment factors, while euphoria was positively correlated with cognitive impairment. This would suggest that early in the onset of cognitive impairment there is a degree of awareness that can often lead to reactive depression. As the impairment progresses and expands, the increasing loss of insight leads to a blissful unawareness and failure to appreciate the sorry circumstances of their condition. Support for such a view can also be gleaned from Reifler and colleagues' study (1982), mentioned earlier in the chapter.

However, the 'paranoid' factor in Gustafson and Hagberg's study seemed quite independent of cognitive impairment, and it is noteworthy that such symptomatology is also identified as a distinct feature in both Jonsson's and Ballinger's studies (Jonsson *et al.*, 1973; Ballinger *et al.*, 1982). Unfortunately, it remains to be seen what external associations can be found to validate the separation of a 'paranoid' or 'paranoid-hallucinating' subtype within dementia, and what future consequences regarding prognosis and response to treatment such a subtyping would result in.

Of more interest at present are the attempts to develop clinical subgroups according to the type of cognitive pathology shown in dementia, and to relate these to underlying neuropathological variations and presumptive aetiologies. Thus there is interest in developing clinical syndrome pictures corresponding, in early dementia, to Alzheimer's, Pick's and multiple infarct dementias; secondly, there is interest in identifying a parieto-temporal deficit syndrome within senile dementia, as representing a more malignant variant of this condition. The attempt to map out discrete cognitive-neuropathological syndromes within dementia is to some extent simply the elaboration of the clinical signs associated with neuropathologically discrete types of cerebral atrophy. Whether or not there are corresponding clinical syndromes associated with discrete neuropathological syndromes is of course of no relevance to the aetiological investigation of these syndromes. It is of more relevance that there are vascular and non-vascular origins to cerebral atrophy in old age, than whether or not certain clinical features, such as confusion of diurnal arousal rhythms, are always associated with the former and not with the latter. Similarly, differentiating the cognitive deficits in Huntington's chorea from Alzheimer's disease is less important than demonstrating the nature of the genetic abnormality in the former. In many ways, one might wish to argue that it is the accompaniments or prodromal signs of the dementia that are of more distinctive relevance to the understanding of these neuropathological conditions, and that the dementia is the common clinical core, reflecting the end-point of cortical atrophy that all these conditions share.

This latter point is, however, not resolved. Several studies have examined clinical and cognitive features of diagnostically discrete groups of (usually pre-senile) dementing patients (Birkett, 1972; Perez *et al.*, 1975; Aminoff *et al.*, 1975; Harrison *et al.*, 1979; Gustafson and Nilsson, 1982). The results have not all been successful. Thus Birkett (1972) found no clear-cut emotional, behavioural or cognitive grounds for separating autopsy-confirmed cerebrovascular dementias from primary atrophy dementia; Harrison *et al.* (1979) found a good separation of CVD from others using Hachinski's Ischemic Scale (Hachinski *et al.*, 1975), though Gustafson and Nilsson (1982) felt it had 'certain limitations'. The studies by Perez *et al.* (1975) and Aminoff *et al.* (1975) both produced differences between groups, but no evidence of discrete patterns of cognitive deficits, on psychometric testing. The separation of Pick's from Alzheimer's dementia was by no means perfect in Gustafson and Nilsson's (1982) study.

There is clearly little evidence that any unique set of cognitive, emotional and behavioural features distinguish between the major pre-senile dementias – notably Alzheimer's, Pick's Huntington's and multiple infarct cerebrovascular dementias. The choreiform movements and family history in Huntington's dementia and the presence of extra-cerebral vascular pathology and a history of cerebrovascular accidents in MID are probably more reliable discriminating clinical features in the latter two conditions than any cognitive, emotional or behavioural signs. However, in discriminating between Pick's and Alzheimer's disease, it may be that certain features of cognitive performance are of interest and value, as indicating differing clinical forms of dementia. These are in particular the differential personality changes, the presence versus absence of spatial orientation and body schema deficits. Table 2.2, derived from Gustafson and Nilsson's report, indicates some of the uniquely differential features.

Table 2.2: Clinical Features Differentially Associated with Alzheimer's and Pick's Dementia

Clinical features	Alzheimer	Pick
Early amnesia for remote events	+	−
Early spatial disorientation	+	−
Apraxia, aphasic and agnosic signs	+	−
Confabulation	−	+
Early signs of disinhibition	−	+
Echolalia, mutism and aminia	−	+

Source: Derived from Gustafson and Nilsson (1982), table 3.

Perhaps the most interesting difference between the two clinical syndromes suggested here is the constrast between focal deficits of established skills (language deficits, deficits of motor execution skills, for example, in handling tools, deficits in spatial orientation, both in relation to finding one's way around, and recalling direction – loss of spatial memory and positional sense, in terms of retention of body image) characterising early Alzheimer's disease and the sustained motor skills, spatial orientation and memory characterising early Pick's dementia, where disinhibition, loss of intentionality and confabulation indicate a more noticeable personality change, often overshadowing the loss of intellectual ability. To some extent this dichotomy – cognitive deficits versus motivational and behavioural anomalies – underlies much of the principal variation in presentation of dementia, irrespective of the neuropathological diagnosis, and as such represents a very different effect on family and neighbours' reactions to the early stages of a person's dementia.

In contrast to attempts primarily focusing upon differentiating between the pre-senile dementia pathologies, recent interest has arisen regarding the extent of variation between the most common pre-senile dementia, Alzheimer's dementia and senile dementia, both of which demonstrate indistinguishable neuropathology (Rossor, 1982). It has been argued that dementia of early onset is more often characterised by marked losses of crystallised skills, such as aphasia and apraxia, which German writers have termed '*Werkzeugstorungen*' (Lauter and Meyer, 1968). Late-age dementias, in contrast, are considered to show fewer such signs, and to follow a slower and smoother cognitive decline, capable of merging into a benign senescence (Kral, 1962). Evidence for such hetero- geneity within the dementias of old age has come from a number of sources. McDonald (1969) observed that within an elderly dement- ing population, a relatively younger group could be identified demonstrating signs of parietal lobe dysfunction (impaired tactile recognition, confusion of left and right, impaired ability to handle and construct simple objects and copy simple shapes) who showed a higher mortality rate. Kasniak *et al.* (1978) also found that early mortality in dementia was associated with tempero-parietal deficits (i.e. language disturbance, disturbed left–right orientation), as did Naguib and Levy (1982). Such findings suggest that when some cognitive losses emerge 'ahead of time' in dementia (i.e. gross impairment of crystallised cognitive skills, without a level of severe overall incompetence), they carry a more severe prognosis than when the decline is more similar to 'normal ageing', with the assumptions of a slower and more measured deterioration.

Unfortunately there is a lack of careful longitudinal investigation in dementia so that such cross-sectional findings, usually based upon institutionalised samples, remain unverified as unique pathways in the dementing process. Many attempts to stage the common path- way in dementia clinically are equally questionable, since they too have been developed from cross-sectional information.

Staging the Pathway of Dementias

One of the most comprehensive attempts to delineate the course of cognitive decline in dementia has recently been described by Reisberg and his colleagues from the New York University Medical Center. They argue that the cognitive decline in dementia 'is a unique clinical syndrome with a characteristic onset and progres- sion' (Reisberg *et al.,* 1982). There are, these writers suggest, three major clinical phases apparent in dementia: an early phase of forgetfulness, when the deficit is principally subjectively noted, though verifiable in cognitive (memory) testing; this is followed by an intermediate, confusional phase, when cognitive deficits are readily apparent to an observer; and finally a late 'dementia' phase, which indicates the onset of sufficient impairment to render in- dependent existence impossible. These three phases are further subdivided into seven stages of decline (though the first stage is one of normality, which is thus irrelevant). The subsequent six stages are briefly described in Table 2.3.

This schematic outline of the progress of dementia has been developed from examination of many hundreds of patients, but it is derived essentially from a cross-sectional understanding of dementia, rather than the following-through of people from the beginning of their dementia to the ultimate end in the vegetative state preceding death. A similar stage model had earlier been described by the Swedish workers, Hagberg, Gustafson and others, in their attempt to classify differing degrees of dementia with onset in middle life. They identified five groups of patients which 'in all likelihood represent successive stages of increasing intellectual reduction in progressive organic dementia' (Hagberg and Ingvar, 1976). While bearing a broad similarity to the above stages, they also postulate that separate patterns of focal impairments can be identified within the context of an overall progressive reduction of intellectual efficiency – in other words, suggesting that variations in the pattern of impairments in established cognitive skills provide for a degree of heterogeneity in dementia, in contrast to the uniformity indicated by Reisberg and his colleagues.

Deducing syndrome patterns and identifying pathways of cognitive decline from cross-sectional sampling of patients may lead to confusion between stages and syndromes. Without longitudinal research, the temporal gradient in dementia cannot be identified. Variations may exist not in how cognitive functions decline, but how quickly they decline, or how quickly deficits emerge. Such variation in rate of impairment may, in turn, facilitate or impede compensatory strategies. Thus the reported confabulation of Pick's dementia may arise because of the milder degree of memory and intellectual decline which permits such compensating behaviour, or alternatively because of a lack of judgement and insight which lets the individual make up unconvincing explanations of forgotten events. To link the deficits and inefficiencies in mental performance to purely endogenously developing atrophic processes is to ignore the complication of brain function, and the limitation of a narrow localisation of function which many neuropsychologists have criticised (Luria, 1973).

Table 2.3: Stage Model of Dementia

Stage		Clinical features	Mental status questionnaire/
Very mild cognitive decline	(1)	Subjective complaints of forgetfulness, especially names and where familiar objects have been placed	No errors
	(2)	No observable deficits in interview, or other social situation	
	(3)	Memory tests reveal below normal performance	
Mild cognitive decline	(1)	Word and name-finding difficulties	No errors
	(2)	Anxiety about memory lapses	
	(3)	May get seriously lost in unfamiliar surroundings	
	(4)	Memory tests reveal abnormal learning impairment	
Moderate cognitive decline	(1)	Decreased knowledge of recent personal and current events	3 or more errors
	(2)	Deficits evident in a number of circumstances	
	(3)	Withdrawal and emotional flattening, with denial of problems	
	(4)	Complex tasks poorly and inaccurately performed (e.g. use of tools)	
Moderately severe cognitive decline	(1)	Disorientation evident in time and often place	4 – 5 errors
	(2)	Occasionally mixed up while getting dressed	
	(3)	Major gaps in knowledge of past and present life circumstances	
Severe cognitive decline	(1)	Largely unaware of current events, experiences and surroundings	5 – 10 errors
	(2)	Incontinence and impaired self-care	
	(3)	Personality changes, including delusional beliefs, obsessional symptoms, agitation, or aggression, and cognitive abulia (loss of intentionality)	

Table 2.3: Stage Model of Dementia (*continued*)

Stage	Clinical features	Mental status questionnaire*
Very severe cognitive decline	(1) Gross impairment of language use and compre- hension (2) Help required in toiletting and dressing (3) Generalised and focal neurological signs present	10 errors

Note: *As compiled by R.L. Kahn *et al.* (1960).
Source: After Reisberg *et al.* (1982).

Overview

Dementia as a clinical syndrome represents a progressive deterioration in all areas of brain function which maintain the individual's
links with his present and past personal, social and physical environment. The reactions and adaptations to such an erosion of the
boundaries of the self provide additional psychopathological
features which may at times, especially early on, overshadow the
original cognitive impairment. As the remaining cognitive self-
maintenance skills decline, so these reactions and adaptations
themselves deteriorate and fail, leading to increasingly regressive
elements in behaviour which bring into sharper focus the extent of
mental incompetence, until the brain ceases to manifest any sustained control over the immediate personal environment and the
person can no longer look after himself. From this point on,
sequences of behaviour become increasingly severed from any sustained, purposive, intact behaviour, eventually resulting in ever-
limited reactivity to the immediate physical environment.
   At one level, then, this deteriorative process begins with a reduction in cognitive or conceptual mastery: new information cannot be
assimilated, and interests and concerns become narrower, more
limited and more concrete. Indifference, dislike or fear of the new
and personally distant world may produce withdrawal, lack of
curiosity and increasing rigidity. Such a retrenchment may be slowly
and apparently successfully negotiated, without evident distress
and with the appearance of retained personal integrity, albeit of a
more egotistical and restricted nature. Alternatively, the inability

to assimilate new or personally distant information may arise more rapidly, resulting in increased threat, especially if the individual's personal and social environment is relatively extensive, where their limited competence can be more severely taxed. As failure in recall and incompetent retrieval strategies become evident, the field of mastery is further reduced, and the immediate familiar environment no longer provides a secure field in which the person can maintain their integrity. At this point, there may be further withdrawal and indifference – to household chores, to family news, etc. – or the employment of evidently incompetent defence mechanisms of denial and projection. As the person shows increasing inability to rationalise effectively, to give plausible accounts of his or her own actions, to relate his or her behaviour to the immediate environment, self-neglect becomes evident. A process of alienation from others then seems to emerge. Close family feel they can no longer understand or get through to the dementing person at this stage. From this point, many of the individual problems of hostility, apathy, wandering, even incontinence now are overshadowed by the more central loss – the loss of the person. The demented individual now seems to have become disoriented, not simply to his own surroundings, but to his previous self. Occasional echoes of the self and old habits emerge, but without evident continuity. Behaviour becomes increasingly reactive, purposeless and disjointed. As even this reactivity declines, a vegetative state predominates, with minimal voluntary activity. Such an end-point seems rarely observed in the community, and may be normally reached only when institutional medical care is continuously maintained.

EPIDEMIOLOGY OF DEMENTIA IN THE
COMMUNITY

Prevalence and Incidence

If the term dementia is extended to include all chronic organic brain
syndromes characterised by deterioration in cognitive functioning,
there is considerable consistency in estimates of prevalence and
incidence in elderly populations. One of the more recent reviews of
this area calculated a likely prevalence rate of 6.5 per cent amongst
the over-65s, for moderate to severe dementia (Kay and Bergmann,
1980). Within the elderly population, there is an associated increase
in prevalence rates which suggests an increasing incidence in
extreme old age, as is demonstrated in Table 3.1.

Table 3.1: Prevalence of Dementia by Age and Sex (percentages)

Age	Males	Females	Overall
65 – 69	3.9	0.5	2.1
70 – 74	4.1	2.7	3.3
75 – 79	8.0	7.9	8.0
80 +	13.2	20.9	17.7

Source: From Kay and Bergmann, 1980, p.43.

Studies such as those by Helgason (1977), on the total Icelandic
population, confirm this accelerative incidence of dementia in
extreme old age, as Table 3.2 shows.

Table 3.2: Incidence (rate per 1000 per year) of Organic Brain
Syndrome in Over-65s

Age	Male	Female
65–69	1.3	0.8
70–74	2.1	2.1
75–79	3.4	4.0
80+	9.4	8.3

Source: From Helgason, 1977.

This population study suggests an almost tenfold increase in the
annual incidence of dementia/organic brain syndrome from age 65 –

69 to the over-80s. In order to place such figures in context, it is helpful to consider the numbers involved in a given age population. Thus estimates of population change between 1961 and 2001 in Britain as a whole are given in Table 3.3.

Table 3.3: Estimates of Population Change in Britain between 1961 and 2001

Age	1961	2001
65–74	4.0m	4.5m
75+	2.1m	3.7m

Source: OPCS (1983).

It can be seen that there will have been a 76 per cent increase in the over-75s, 10 per cent of whom can be assumed to suffer dementing illnesses, in contrast to a 12 per cent increase in the young elderly (65 – 74), with a 2.5 per cent prevalence of dementia. This will result in approximately 175,000 additional cases of dementia at the end of a 40-year period, compared with the situation in the early 1960s, when much of the pioneering epidemiological studies of Roth and his colleagues at Newcastle were carried out. This is almost equivalent to the total elderly population in all types of residential care in the UK in 1979 (177,400).

It is well known that the majority of elderly patients suffering from dementia live in the community. Kay and Bergmann (1980) suggest that between 20 per cent and 25 per cent of the moderately and severely demented are living in institutional care. Helgason (1977) found that although 25 per cent of elderly patients with severe organic brain syndromes came to the attention of the psychiatric services in Iceland, only 10 per cent of those with less than severe syndromes did so. This underlines the as yet unattended problems of the mildly or questionably dementing elderly population.

Living Circumstances

There is little detailed information on the social and living circumstances of the dementing elderly in the community. One of the earliest surveys in Britain was carried out by Kay, Beamish and Roth (1964). They found no social-class or marital-status differences between dementing and non-dementing persons in the community, nor for the women were there significant differences in the numbers living alone. However, it is apparent that whilst 24 per cent of the normal male elderly and 29 per cent of the normal female elderly lived alone, none of the dementing males ($n = 14$) and 53 per cent of the dementing females ($n = 15$) lived alone. From these small numbers it is difficult to generalise, yet it does seem that it is rare for the elderly male dementing patient to live alone in the community, but not uncommon for the elderly female dementing patient to do so.

Bergmann *et al.* (1978) found that of 83 consecutive referrals to a geriatric psychiatry assessment service, 38 per cent lived alone, 34 per cent with their children, and 26 per cent with their spouse only. Bond and Carstairs (1982) examined the living arrangements of a large community sample of over-65s in Clackmannan, and found that 48 per cent of those with mild dementia and 42 per cent of those with severe dementia were living alone. Some 16 per cent of the former and 13 per cent of the latter lived with spouses only, while 35 per cent and 45 per cent respectively lived with others (mostly children or siblings).

Gaspar (1980) in a survey of 230 referrals to a psychiatric dementia service also found differences in living arrangements between male and female patients. While only 16 per cent of the male dementia patients lived alone, 33 per cent of the female patients did so. In contrast, 56 per cent of the male patients lived with their spouse, but only 26 per cent of the female patients did so. However, it is likely that these figures simply reflect national demographic trends; for example, 1979/80 General Household Survey returns indicate that 17 per cent of elderly males live alone, whereas 45 per cent of elderly females do so. Likewise, over 70 per cent of elderly males live with their spouse, in constrast to 37 per cent of the women (61 per cent and 32 per cent respectively living with spouse only).

In conclusion, data on living arrangements of the dementing elderly in the community seem to reflect general demographic patterns. Elderly males are usually living with a spouse, whereas elderly females are equally found to be living alone, living with a spouse, or living with others (children, siblings, etc.).

The significance of living arrangements has been pointed out in Bergmann's (1978) study. While 18.5 per cent of those dementing elderly patients living alone survived for one year in the community,

40 per cent of those living with supporters did so. Gaspar's (1980) study, however, suggests additional sex influences on community outcome: over the two-year period, he found that 63 per cent of the dementing males entered long-term care, in contrast to 40 per cent of the women. One may conclude that living with a supporter is a less 'protective' factor against institutional care for men than it is for women. This may well be that men are less easily managed at home, perhaps because of their greater potential for aggression and abusive behaviour. Finally, in a recent Japanese study, involving a five-year follow-up of dementia patients, Hasegawa and Homma (1981) found 'that at least in intermediate terms there is actually no difference of mortality rate between the institutionalised aged and the community resident aged [dementing patients]'. The implication of no gross environmental effects on mortality rates of the elderly mentally infirm has also been noted in two British studies (Gilleard and Pattie, 1978; MacDonald *et al.*, 1982).

Mortality and Dementia

Studies examining the survival times of individuals suffering from dementia are quite rare. While several studies have examined mortality figures of patients admitted to hospital with a diagnosis of dementia, most of the values derive from 'time of admission' to subsequent death (Roth, 1955; Larsson, Sjogren and Jacobson, 1963; Shah, Banks and Merskey, 1969; Thompson and Eastwood, 1981; Christie, 1982). While there is some dispute whether or not post-institutionalisation survival time has increased in recent years (Thompson and Eastwood, 1981; Christie, 1982), the average survival time does seem to be quite consistently around two years. Excluding the significant proportion who die within the first year of admission, subsequent average survival time is around two and a half years (Larsson *et al.*, 1963; Shah *et al.*, 1969), which may be the result of patients being admitted to hospital because of additional physical disease, and thus distorting and reducing the natural survival time in dementia.

Since Larsson *et al.* (1963), unlike the other hospital-based studies, also included data on age of onset, it is possible to identify the likely survival time between onset and death – slightly less than five years for men, slightly more than five years for women. A recent study by Heston *et al.* (1981), focusing upon a more carefully delineated sample of patients with 'dementia of the Alzheimer type', mostly derived from autopsy records, observed an average survival time of around seven years (for those with onset after the age of 64). Aside from the discrepancy in these two studies, one common point is that the enhanced mortality, relative to expected survival, declines with increasing age. Thus late-onset dementia (after age 80 years) results in a less discrepant survival rate, whereas early onset (below age 65 years) results in a markedly enhanced mortality.

Swedish mortality figures indicate a mean 18-year life expectation at the age of 60 years; a mean 10-year life expectancy at age 70; a mean 6-year life expectancy at age 80; and a mean 3-year life expectancy at age 90 (cf. Larsson *et al.*, 1963, p. 101; Nielsen, Homma and Biorn-Henrikson, 1977). What may be deduced from these figures is that the expected survival of elderly individuals developing dementia does not greatly differ from that of elderly individuals not developing dementia, unless the onset of mental decline occurs before the age of 75. It is probable that supporters who care for an elderly relative beginning to show signs of mental deterioration may expect, therefore, six to eight years of coping, with ever-increasing problems. Such extended caregiving may involve a gradually increasing burden for family members that may extend beyond their limits to maintain care over such a prolonged period.

Table 3.4: Average Survival Rates for Dementia Patients at Different Ages of Onset

Age of onset	*n*	Larsson *et al.* (1963) Average survival rate (years)	*n*	Heston *et al.* (1981) Average survival rate (years)
<65	20	8.7	63	8.3
65–74	82	6.2	78	8.4
75–84	91	4.5	38	5.9
85 +	15	3.8	9	5.0

Sources: Larsson *et al.* (1963) and Heston *et al.* (1981).

Finally, the issue of 'onset' needs to be raised once more. As Heston *et al.* (1981) remark, clinical estimates are 'in many cases' very crude. Larsson *et al.* (1963), for example, while recognising the 'approximate' nature of their data, provide no criterion for judging onset, while Heston *et al.* (1981) use as a criterion 'the age at which failure to remember new information first becomes irreversibly established'. However, what constitutes 'failure to remember' is problematic – viz. Kral's 'benign memory loss' in old age (Kral, 1962). At least one-third, maybe half, of 'questionable dementias' identified in epidemiological studies may fail to dement progressively (Bergmann *et al.*, 1971). Clearly, there is still little hard information to give to a relative who asks 'how long will this go on?' Until sufficiently careful prospective studies of the course of dementia have been made, there can only be very approximate information for carers to go on.

Epidemiology of Support

Marital status and living arrangements give only a crude picture of the nature of support given to dementing elderly in the community. Kay *et al.* (1964) found that their dementing sample were relatively less well off for amenities in the home, and had a more restricted level of daily social contacts, compared with both normal elderly people, and those with non-organic psychiatric disorders. Contact with children (numbers not seeing children weekly or more often) and with siblings (numbers not seeing siblings monthly or more often) did not, however, distinguish their group of dementia patients from the other elderly groups, nor were they less likely to have surviving children or siblings. It would seem that any lack of social/family support observed for such individuals is a function again of overall patterns of support given the elderly. However, one may well have expected *more* contact for such individuals, given their likely greater need for help.

Bond and Carstairs (1982) in their Clackmannan study found that total contacts of the dependent elderly were 'no different to those of other groups', while 'the small group with severe mental impairment had fewer outside social contacts than other groups'. This would point to a pattern of greater reliance upon contacts from the home/family and relative isolation from a wider social network amongst the elderly mentally impaired, and one may consequently assume a greater demand placed upon the home/family of such persons.

Summary

A moderate to severe degree of dementia can be observed in one out of every 15 people over the age of 65, and in one out of every 10 over the age of 75. The development of a new case of dementia will occur for every 100 people over 80, each year.

In Britain, at least, the majority of such people will be living in private households, and will have very similar social characteristics to the elderly in general; that is, the men will rarely be living alone, while the women will, in over one-third of cases, be on their own. Regular family contact will be the rule, not the exception.

Close kin (spouses, siblings, children) are as likely to be in contact with dementing elderly people as they are in the general population, but there will be less contact with others outside this primary kinship network. Formal services will be received by more of the dementing elderly than is the case for the general elderly adult population.

Those caring for the elderly mentally infirm, mostly children or spouses, will on average experience six to eight years when mental decline of their relative is evident. Since hospitalisation or other institutional care is a likely outcome for those living alone, such people seem likely to be managed for four to five years in independent households before admission to care. Obviously these figures are average ones, but they do indicate that even for those dementing elderly who do enter institutional settings, the major part of their illness will have been spent in the community.

4 COMMUNITY SERVICES FOR THE ELDERLY MENTALLY INFIRM: CURRENT LEVELS OF PROVISION

Many countries, North America in particular, single Britain out as the forerunner in the provision of community services to the elderly, and particularly the elderly infirm. It is perhaps the result of Britain being slower in expanding alternative residential accommodation for such a population that this historical emphasis on community care has developed. This relative under-provision of institutional services is evident in international comparisons of residential provision for the elderly. As an example, Table 4.1 illustrates how some other European countries compare with Britain in making provisions for their elderly population.

Table 4.1: Over-65s in Institutional or Sheltered Care, European Variations (rates per 1,000 over 65)

	Netherlands	Denmark	Sweden	Scotland	England
Sheltered housing	86.7	50.6	31.6	12.0	26.0
Residential homes	116.7 ⎱	70 ⎱	50.0	18.0	18.5
Nursing homes	16.7 ⎰	82 ⎰	33.3	—	—
Hospital	—			13.3	8.5
Overall level of institutional provision	133.4	78.2	83.3	31.3	27.0

Source: Thom (1981), table 2.3, p. 39.

When the receipt by the elderly of institutional care is examined in more detail, it is apparent that the use of institutional resources increases exponentially for the older old-age groups in the population. Table 4.2 illustrates this phenomenon, employing data from the 1971 United Kingdom census, and comparative data derived from a provincial census in Sweden, undertaken in 1975 (Adolfsson et al., 1981).

While the level of provision is clearly greater in Sweden, both countries demonstrate that it is the over-80s who are most likely to receive institutional care, and of course, it is in this age-group that the prevalence of dementia or chronic brain syndrome is greatest.

Table 4.2: Age and Institutional Care: a Comparison between Two European Countries of Percentage in Care

Age	UK	Sweden
65–69	2.5	2.0
70–74	3.9	5.0
75–79	6.4	13.0
80–84	11.8	27.0
85–89	19.2	47.0
90+	30.0	70.0

Sources: UK population census, 1971 and Adolfsson *et al.* (1981).

According to one recent survey, approximately 50 per cent of residents in old people's homes, 65 per cent of residents in geriatric hospitals, and more than 90 per cent of residents in psychogeriatric hospital wards are 'confused' (Charlesworth and Wilkin, 1982). Thus, although dementia remains more prevalent in the community, as the previous chapter showed, in absolute numbers it still accounts for the majority of institutional beds in Britain. Because of the ageing of the over-65-year-old population, there has been a need to expand the number of residential places available to the elderly. Equally, there has been an increase in the provision of community-based health and personal social services. Figures from Scotland illustrate this trend (see Table 4.3).

Similar data and trends are evident in England and Wales (Bebbington, 1979; Grundy and Arie, 1982). What is most apparent is that while residential-care provision has not effectively kept pace with the rise in the over-75-year-old population, domiciliary and day-care services have expanded at a much faster rate, especially within the personal social services sector, reaching out to a greater proportion of the elderly over the last decade.

These trends in expanding community services can be seen as governmental and societal responses to helping maintain the elderly in their own homes; the question arises regarding the extent to which such services meet the needs of the elderly mentally infirm and their families. In order to examine this question it is helpful to examine the current level of receipt of such services by the over-65-year-old population. Data from the General Household Surveys of 1980 and 1981 provide a useful index of the current level of provision (see Table 4.4).

Given this baseline level of service provision, how well do the elderly mentally infirm do as recipients of such services? Few surveys of the elderly mentally infirm have provided sufficient

Table 4.3: Trends in Institutional and Community Service Provision to the Over-65s in Scotland

	1973	1976	1979	1981	Percentage increase 1973–81
No. of old people's homes	222	236	244	249	10.8
No. of beds	7,982	8,216	8,745	8,845	10.8
Home nursing cases aged over 65 (000s)	85.9	89.8	100.5	108.1	25.8
Health visitor cases aged over 65 (000s)	84.0	90.6	96.3	101.7	21.1
Home helps	36.4	59.2	71.5	78.8	116.5
No. of households visited (over-65s) (000s)					
Meals-on-wheels	14.5	14.1	13.2	14.6	0.7
No. of day care centres	12	36	49	52	
No. of places for over 65s	1,833	2,800	3,329	4,500	145.5
Population					
85 +	39,100	41,200	42,950	47,620	21.8
75 +	226,300	241,600	259,900	275,860	21.9
65 +	669,000	698,000	717,700	737,750	10.3

Source: Scottish Abstract of Statistics, 1973–1981.

Table 4.4: Current Patterns of Use by the Over-65s of Community Health Services and Personal Social Services, Occurring in the Last Month (percentage)

Community health service	1980	1981
Visited GP at surgery	27	24
GP visited at home	11	10
Seen district nurse or health visitor	6	6
Chiropodist	11	10
Home help	9	9
Meals-on-wheels	2	3
Day centre	5	5

Source: General Household Surveys, 1980 and 1981.

information to make direct comparisons. Bond and Carstairs (1982) in their survey of the elderly population in Clackmannan identified a group of mentally impaired elderly, whom they subdivided into ambulant and non-ambulant categories. Table 4.5 shows the service received by these groups, contrasted with the base population.

Table 4.5: Services Received by Elderly Mentally Infirm, Clackmannan Survey

Service	Mentally impaired, ambulant	Mentally impaired, non-ambulant	Base
District nurse	4.2	50.0	6.2
Health visitor	12.5	5.6	3.0
Home help	20.0	33.3	11.1
Meals-on-wheels	12.5	8.3	3.2

Source: Bond and Carstairs (1982).

An earlier study, described in full by Isaacs, Neville and Livingston (1972), reported on the services received by a sample of elderly patients before they were admitted for geriatric inpatient care: in their 'mentally abnormal' subsample, 19 per cent received home helps and 26 per cent visits from the district nurse. In our own survey of referrals to psychogeriatric day care (to be described in more detail later), 34 per cent were visited by either a district nurse or less commonly, a health visitor, 32 per cent had home helps and 10 per cent meals-on-wheels. All these surveys point to the likelihood that the elderly with significant mental infirmity are more likely to receive community health and social services than the average elderly person, confirming the findings of the earlier community survey conducted in Newcastle (Foster, Kay and Bergmann, 1976). What both the Clackmannan survey and the Newcastle survey also show is that the combination of both physical infirmity and mental impairment is likely to draw the greatest amount of support from these services, raising the question of the adequacy of service provision to the physically fit dementing group living in the community.

Before turning from this broad overview of community service provision to concentrate on the role played by each service in more detail, it should be pointed out just how variable service provisions are between districts, areas and regions. Vetter, Jones and Victor (1981) in their study of such variation in the Welsh counties observed that in some counties almost 40 per cent of the elderly were seen by district nurses, while in others only 14 per cent were seen: similar variations, not quite so marked, occurred for home helps, meals-on-wheels and health visitors. Variations in level of provision have also been noted by Gruer (1975) in the Scottish Borders, and doubtless other regions would produce similar disparities in service provision. As a result, it is necessary to exercise caution in interpreting broad national trends in the development of community services to each particular locality.

Community Health Services

Apart from the doctor, community health care resides in the hands of the district nurse and health visitor. As Table 4.3 shows, the increase in visits made by both these professional groups has surpassed the growth in the elderly population overall, though the increase simply parallels the increase in the over-75 age-groups. Nearly all surveys demonstrate quite clearly that the very old and those with disability are considerably more likely to receive such services. For example, the General Household Survey, 1981, indicates that while only 3 per cent of those aged 65 – 69 years receive visits, 27 per cent of those aged 85 years and over do so. Even so, substantial numbers of elderly infirm, and particularly the elderly fit, but mentally infirm group, do not receive visits from either home nurses or health visitors.

It is important to recognise the likely differences in involvement associated with health visiting and home nursing. While district nurses can be seen as having a practical 'hands-on' service, helping with bathing, dressings, bed making, skin care, enemas, and other treatment interventions, this role operates very much at the level of physical care and physical disabilities. It is not surprising to find that higher proportions of the geriatric mentally infirm receive, and probably benefit from, district nurse visits than is the case with the fit but dementing elderly person, whose needs differ substantially from those currently met by the district nursing service. Health visitors are seen as having a less directly caregiving role than district nurses, and almost as a consequence have a less clear-cut job to do. Luker (1981), discussing the role of the health visitor in community care, reports an observational study of health visiting practice which she carried out, and which indicated that 'visits to the elderly were unstructured and seemed to have no plan at all'. She argues that the low priority given by health visitors to visiting the elderly (Clark, 1981, found on average only 17.5 per cent of visits were to the elderly) results from their having 'no useful frame of reference from which to make a meaningful, relevant and satisfying contribution' (Luker, 1981).

Surveillance and screening of elderly populations have been widely advocated as a suitable role for the health visitor, and a good case can be made for providing this alternative to 'demand-based care' for the elderly infirm. However, studies evaluating the effectiveness of such screening services have not found strong evidence of improved health and competence resulting from such surveillance (Tulloch and Moore, 1979; Barber and Wallis, 1978).

This problem is especially relevant to an elderly mentally infirm population, for whom screening is perhaps especially important. While it is unclear whether community services would improve their disabilities, it is likely to lead to an enhanced service provision (Barber and Wallis, 1982). The question then arises as to how effective an enhanced service provision is. In an important American study of community-care services to the elderly infirm, Blenkner and colleagues (1971) found that the group receiving 'intervention' had, as a consequence, heightened mortality rates and greater levels of institutionalisation. Very few people in Britain are advocating a community-care service that will increase the pressure on institutional beds!

Personal Social Services

Field Social Workers

To a large extent the problems facing health visitors are not unlike those facing the field social worker – namely, those of developing an appropriate frame of reference, and lacking an appropriate back-up structure within the community, to direct and determine the pattern of intervention. Much of social work revolves around a collaborative model of helping. Crosbie (1983) has recently carried out an interesting analysis of the activities of field social workers in dealing with the elderly. While more than 80 per cent of the clients perceived as needing help with mobility problems concurred with the social workers' view, less than 5 per cent of clients considered 'confused' by the social worker shared such a view themselves. This problem of failure to perceive disability is common to the majority of dementing people in the community (Reifler, Cox and Hanley, 1981) and clearly presents difficulties for a collaborative model of care. Much of social-work visiting revolves around arranging aids, home helps and admission to residential care, and is premised upon meeting the expressed needs of the people served. Opit (1977), in a study of elderly infirm people receiving domiciliary services, pointed out that while half of the people were on social-work files, less than 10 per cent were regularly visited by social workers. Obviously, much social work at this level involves office work and liaison, rather than direct counselling, yet, given the frequent limited social network surrounding the elderly mentally infirm, there would seem to be a need for social workers to maintain contacts with such socially fragile community residents.

Recently, indeed, there has been interest in developing a broader role for social work with the elderly, piloted in the Kent community care project (Challis and Davies, 1980). Discussing some of the trends in the population changes and level of residential provision illustrated in Table 4.3, these authors argued: 'The relative contribution of the residential home must therefore be expected to fall dramatically during the next few years, placing greater strain on domiciliary support than in the past. There is a real danger that existing domiciliary services will be unable to meet these rising needs' (Challis and Davies, 1980). In response to this situation, they set up a pilot project giving a small team of social workers the responsibility of developing interlocking care services, supplementary to those currently present, for elderly clients referred to the social services department for residential care. Much of the social workers' task involved enrolling volunteer and other part-time workers to offer a flexible care service, not normally available from the statutory services (e.g. weekend support, help after office hours, etc.). Payment to these volunteers was made to 'remove disincentives to helping, rather than acting as an incentive itself'. By employing a control group of clients also put forward for residential care, but not receiving the supplementary support network developed by the project team, they were able to evaluate the impact of this innovatory service. While the majority of the control group had been institutionalised one year later, clients referred to the experimental service were still mostly surviving in the community.

This 'key-worker' scheme of gathering together support from the community seems to offer a more positive role for social work with the elderly 'at risk', and may be especially suitable for the elderly mentally infirm as a means of providing relief for carers, without undermining the existing supports received.

Home Helps and Meals-on-Wheels

Unlike the care-managing role of health visitors and social workers, the home-help service, like home nursing services, represents a 'hands-on' caregiving system. Overall, one in ten of the over-65-year-old population is likely to receive home help, ranging from 2 per cent of those in their sixties to over 25 per cent of the over-80s. Surveys of the elderly mentally infirm indicate that a similar proportion (20–25 per cent) receive home-help services (Bond and Carstairs, 1982; Isaacs, *et al.*, 1972; Bergmann *et al.*, 1978), though this is mostly directed to those living alone, or with an equally elderly spouse or sibling. The potential benefits of the home-help service for the carers of the elderly mentally infirm extend beyond their direct assistance in domestic work, shopping and physical assistance (for example, in dressing); because they spend between one and one and a half hours at the home, they offer the added benefit of a temporary 'sitting service', allowing the supporter time to go out and escape from the continuous demands of supervision.

One husband described this situation as follows:

I got the home help then [after seeing the social worker] which I didn't think was going to be much good really because I could do all that was necessary, housework and that, and getting her sorted out, I could do all that, but well this one's been for quite a while and it's quite a good thing, that, because I can leave her for two hours when the home help is there, and get out with the dog and maybe do a bit of shopping, and this home help is very understanding, she knows the position . . .

Clearly, such releasing of the need for supervision is a great help to such individuals, and is a unique benefit of the home-help service, with their extended contact time – unlike, for example, the briefer visits of the district nurse, community psychiatric nurse or health visitor. The rising level of provision evident over the last decade clearly will result in more of the elderly at risk receiving a service which many believe sustains more of the infirm elderly at home than does any other community resource. Developments in the home-help service, such as that described by Latto (1981) in Coventry, point the way to a greater integration of the service within social work services, and a more effective role in preventative care. Nevertheless, such schemes remain essentially demonstration projects, waiting for a more widespread application, and a careful appraisal of their specific efficacy with elderly mentally infirm clients. Perhaps the main problem with the service, as far as the elderly mentally infirm and their supporters are concerned, is that adult children living with their dementing parent rarely benefit from this form of relief, and that normally means a daughter who is tied down to a position of constant surveillance.

Meals-on-wheels, reaching a much smaller proportion of the elderly than the home-help service, has not shown any substantial increase over the last eight years in Scotland, nor does it appear to have done so in other parts of Britain. While it may reduce some of the chores of supporters in preparing meals for their dementing relative, it does not provide the sort of service which ensures that the dementing elderly living alone gets a regular meal, and luncheon clubs unfortunately rarely cater for this group.

Day Centres and Day Hospitals

The development of day-care services for the elderly has been a slow process, accelerating most rapidly in the last five or six years. Historically, numerous accounts of the day-hospital movement have been given – in relation to psychiatry (Farndale, 1961) and geriatrics (Brocklehurst, 1970, 1973; Brocklehurst and Tucker, 1980). It is generally recognised that day-hospital care first arose in psychiatry and was then adopted by geriatrics, when the first geriatric day hospital was established in Oxford, in 1952. Despite its origins in psychiatry, the development of specialised psycho-geriatric day hospitals has lagged behind geriatric day hospitals to a quite remarkable extent, and is only now becoming a regular feature of psychogeriatric services.

Day centres, which are usually run by social services/social work departments, are frequently seen as a complementary and overlapping service with day hospitals, and themselves are distinguishable from the luncheon club centres, funded by the local authorities and by voluntary organisations. The history of the day centre for the elderly is less well documented than the day hospital, though it is generally recognised as a recent innovation (Fennell *et al.*, 1981;

Tibbett and Tombs, 1981). The 1981 General Household Survey included an item in its questionnaire for the over-65s, and reported that some 5 per cent of the elderly sampled had been attending day centres for the elderly, figures for geriatric and psychogeriatric day hospitals not being available. Certainly such attendance figures indicate that day centres are a more widespread service than day hospitals, though problems of definition make direct comparisons difficult. Thus in day-services studies carried out in both Scotland and England and Wales, Tibbett and Tombs (1981) and Edwards, Sinclair and Gorbach (1980) describe day units in general as 'a form of communal care which has caregivers present in a non-residential or non-domiciliary setting for at least three days per week, and which is open for at least four hours per day'. Of 13 local authorities sampled in England and Wales, there were 81 day centres, and 42 day hospitals; of the Scottish survey of 80 day units, 57 were day centres and 23 day hospitals. Both studies, conducted in 1978, indicate a ratio of approximately two day centres to one day hospital. Brocklehurst and Tucker (1980) found 102 day centres in the catchment area of two day hospitals.

Day hospitals are obviously health-board funded, whereas day centres are mainly run by social services or voluntary organisations. In 1977, Tibbett and Tombs (1981) found 25 per cent were run purely by social services, while the majority were run by voluntary organisations, often with financial support from local authorities. Provision of day centres may vary widely – for example, in their 1976 survey, Fennell *et al.* (1981) report that within East Anglia, the number of day hospital places for the elderly varied from 3.6 per 1,000 aged over 65 to 10.2 per 1,000 aged over 65; day centre places varied even more, from 2.7 to 13.9 places per 1,000 aged over 65.

To what extent is day care a service provision geared for the elderly mentally infirm? Tibbett and Tombs (1981) found that there were, in Scotland, in 1976, only eight day hospitals (and no day care centres) catering specifically for the elderly mentally infirm – representing approximately 10 per cent of the units set up for the elderly. In a 1970 report, to the SHHD, it was stated that there were only two day hospitals for the elderly mentally infirm in Scotland (SHHD, 1970), so clearly there had been a growth between 1970 and 1977 in levels of provision. In 1982, we conducted a survey of all the Scottish health boards, and found a total of 25 day hospital units for the elderly mentally infirm – indicating an accelerating trend over the decade, and closely paralleling the rise in day centres for the elderly indicated in Table 4.3. Brocklehurst and Tucker (1980) report that in over one-third of the areas including geriatric day hospitals, there was separate day-hospital provision for psycho-geriatric patients, but that in more than half of the areas there was no such provision, nor did the existing geriatric day hospitals accept responsibility for such patients. Indeed, in these latter authors' survey of patients attending 30 day hospitals, only 4 per cent carried a primary diagnosis of dementia, while an additional 5 per cent were also considered to be dementing in the presence of another major illness. Fennell *et al.* (1981), in their survey of day units in East Anglia, found only one day centre which catered for the elderly mentally infirm and 'only one or two confused or senile users are to be found in ordinary day centres' – perhaps the most frequent reason being that they are generally disliked by the other users. These authors quote users who stopped attending a day centre because 'some of them were senile and couldn't talk' or 'some of them are a bit mental' or 'it's like a lunatic asylum there'. Such segregation policies are apparent also in Brocklehurst and Tucker's (1980) survey of staff's views in geriatric day hospitals, who reported that 'staff in almost all day hospitals visited felt that demented patients should be looked after in a different day hos-pital'. Similar findings have been reported in the United States (Kahn and Tobin, 1981).

Clearly, these day hospitals and day centres for the elderly are reluctant to take on the elderly mentally infirm; the dementing elderly person is likely to be served either by psychogeriatric day hospitals or specialised day centres for the elderly mentally infirm, few of which exist. Guidelines laid out for the number of psycho-geriatric places in day hospitals by the DHSS in 1972 were 2.3 per 1,000 of the population aged over 65 years. Surveys of psycho-geriatric day hospitals have not been carried out and it is difficult to ascertain the current level of provision, but indirectly, from studies such as those by Brocklehurst and Tucker (1980) and Tibbett and Tombs (1981), the overall impression is that such facilities are inadequately provided. While some (for example, Whitehead, 1974) have described the day hospital as the centre of the psycho-geriatric service, it is probably equally true to say that many psy-chogeriatric services do not even have a day-hospital service at all. In one study of all psychogeriatric referrals within the Tayside Health Board, during 1974, only 2.8 per cent were directly referred for day care. By 1977, only 15 patients had attended as day-care patients, from 352 patients with a diagnosis of dementia referred to the psychiatric hospitals (that is, 4 per cent of psychiatrically referred demented patients received day care over a three-year period) (Ballinger *et al.*, 1981). Things have improved, but even so, in 1980, a survey of psychogeriatric services indicated that a quarter (22 out of 87) of the services still had no day hospital (Wattis *et al.*, 1981), 70 out of 77 services offered less than two places per 1,000 people aged over 65 in their catchment area, and the majority in fact offered one place per 2,000 or less. As pointed out earlier, an expansion in psychogeriatric day hospitals in Scotland, at least, has taken place during the last decade (1970–1980). Coincidentally, studies are now being reported of the functioning and effectiveness of these services (for example, Greene and Timbury, 1979; Jones and Munbodh, 1982; MacDonald *et al.*, 1982). The results of these studies do not provide strong evidence for the effectiveness of day-hospital care for the elderly mentally infirm as an alternative to institutional care; both Green and Timbury (1979) and Jones and Munbodh (1982) found that by six months the majority of patients were admitted to institutions or had died. MacDonald *et al.*, (1982) found that for a group of matched mild-to-moderately impaired elderly dementing patients, outcome was more favourable if they attended day centres than if they were in institutional care or attended day hospital.

The problems of evaluating day-hospital services for the elderly mentally infirm are numerous; some of the different and indeed conflicting demands on the services, and notions of what it should be, are illustrated in Smith's (1982) paper, describing one set of approaches towards evaluation of such units. What happens inside the day hospital and how effective it is seen to be (and indeed how important it is within the context of the total pattern of services available) are by no means congruent. The particular mix of activities may be described as offering recreation, stimulation, advice, physical care and nutrition – in varying combinations. The evident trend is for places to be increasingly offered to the cognitively impaired elderly, with a varying minority of patients with social and emotional problems often attending on separate days, when there is added group therapy and problem-solving groups. In some cases, speech therapy and physiotherapy may be available to selected patients, but the bulk of activities are controlled by nursing and occupational therapy staff.

Tibbett and Tombs (1981) found that 'bingo was almost universal' in day hospitals (though not in day centres), arts and crafts (knitting, sewing, toy-making, ceramics, painting and canework), and physical treatment (medication, chiropody, special treatments – enemas, baths, dressings, injections, etc.). In day hospitals for the elderly with mental disability, group meetings were 'in some instances an integral part of the programme', as also were reality-orientation groups and other memory games (e.g. the 'Recall' programme, produced by Age Concern). Domestic activities (cooking, baking, washing-up) are also a frequent element of the psychogeriatric day hospital programme, and increasingly use is being made of relatives' group meetings, when family members can discuss some of the problems they face in caring for their elderly mentally impaired relative (cf. Watt, 1982).

Summary

The present chapter may be summarised as follows. There exists a potentially wide range of community services available to the elderly in the community that could, on paper, be seen as meeting most of the needs of those experiencing difficulty in caring for an elderly mentally infirm relative. Such services are, moreover, most often directed to those obviously in need (the old, those living alone, the housebound, non-ambulant elderly person). While community health services have essentially kept pace with the growth in the over-75-year-old age-group, personal social services have shown signs of an increasing level of provision.

At the same time, the situation of the carer of the elderly mentally infirm is in some ways not the centre of this focus of need. Mobility and physical incapacity may not be serious problems for such patients, there may not be major physical needs, in either the sense of nursing or domestic aid, and, of course, the elderly mentally infirm person may be living in a family household. Under these circumstances, the principal need may be to ease the demand of caring, worrying over risks, and having to persuade someone to carry out self-care tasks which may be resisted or misinterpreted by the elderly person whose awareness of difficulties may be blunted or absent. It is one thing to give a bed bath to an elderly isolated and frail lady who appreciates both the physical and emotional contact of a familiar, if not family, face. But to try and persuade a severely confused elderly person to bathe when they believe they are being burned, drowned, or have already had a bath, is considerably less rewarding, and less easily fitted into the regular services of the community nurse.

Day care, as a means of providing relief for the carer, clearly offers an alternative, but it still leaves four or five days each week, and seven nights, when the supporter is left alone with the problems – and it may represent a relief of only five or six hours two days a week. Distress about entering the ambulance, refusal to get ready, and a failure to appreciate where one is being taken can, in some cases, lead to an abandonment of day care, while at an early stage the patient may be so put off by the interaction with more advanced cases that they too cease to attend. Furthermore, day-care provision for the elderly may specifically exclude the elderly mentally infirm, and limit the access of such people to a still relatively small number of psychogeriatric day hospitals and day centres for the elderly mentally infirm.

There is, in Britain, enormous variation in provision of services; some local authorities are 'well off' for home helps, meals-on-wheels, others are well off with district nurses and community psychiatric nurses, while others have little of either. The use of night nursing services is one useful development of value to dementing patients and their relatives (Gillespie, 1980), but is not by any means widely available. Day centres specialising in work with the elderly mentally impaired are another recent development, and may indeed be more acceptable than day hospitals attached to well-known mental hospitals, but again they are rarities rather than regular features of community service resources (Fennell *et al.*, 1981). Psychogeriatric day care may in some areas be fairly well developed and contribute significantly to the numbers of elderly mentally impaired receiving expert psychiatric care, although in other areas it may be completely non-existent.

Not only are there questions of variation in provision and appropriateness of service need, but there is the further issue of integration of community services. The major division between the health service structure of command and accountability and that of the social services is often bemoaned, with workers in both fields criticising the lack of communication with each other. Yet even within these two services there are sufficient communication problems to further complicate a sensitive caring service. Day hospitals grew out of hospital services and relate very much as hospital departments to the primary health-care team, with the result that very few GPs or home nurses from the practice visit or spend time with the day hospital team, who may be linked with a psychogeriatric team largely concerned with inpatient waiting lists and hospital laundry services.

It is ironic that Britain is seen, in both North America and the rest of Europe, as a country pioneering in community services to the elderly, and yet is still incapable of drawing together these many pioneering acts into a genuinely comprehensive and caring system for the elderly mentally infirm. Perhaps because of the general efficiency of geriatric health care, we have developed too similar an approach in psychogeriatrics, drawing upon similar resources and strategies, but by doing so we have failed to identify accurately the problems the community faces with its elderly mentally infirm citizens. It is those problems that the next chapter addresses.

5 DEMENTIA IN THE HOME: PROBLEMS FACED BY CAREGIVERS

Development and Definition of Problems

As has been mentioned, the development of dementia may be an insidious process, causing unease and uncertainty in those supporters living with the elderly person. Trying to cope with the early problems involves the added strain of wondering what the matter is, what is happening to their dependant. Behavioural disturbance and disability do not emerge fully-fledged as problems, but rather evolve from minor oddities and lapses. Sometimes these problems only show themselves in the home, and the dementing individual retains an appearance of complete normality to visitors and neighbours. One woman said of her husband: 'He's like Jekyll and Hyde: I get all the abuse, but people outside, that he meets, he'll be just quite polite and everything, but anything he seemed to want to get off his mind, I get it.' The problem is not just one of abusiveness; it is the selective nature of the abuse, the feeling that others outside the home cannot see what is going on.

This pattern of evolving problems, adaptations, then further new problems requiring further new adjustments itself produces a cycle of continuing strain which slowly wears tolerance away. One husband, describing the onset and development of incontinence in his wife, illustrates the difficulties:

> This incontinence was a gradual process, because she used to get up through the night, about twice she used to go to the bathroom, and then sometimes she used to not be able to get to the bathroom in time, she got caught short, on the floor, and sometimes on the bed. So then I got rubber sheets, for the bed, and I got a commode as well, which she used, she did get up and use the commode. That was all right, that was that sort of problem over, but then eventually, she didn't . . . it was the bed that got wet. I had to get pads after that, and that was another problem, I had to get pads on her . . . and now, I don't really know, I just take it she just doesn't know, because now there are bowel movements as well, and I have to clean up, and of course I get annoyed, naturally, but she, she swears that she never did it, even in the

bed, she says it could have been animals or something . . . *"Problems"*

Often the problems mount up, so that the supporter has little time to reflect upon what is happening, and simply soldiers on through each day, with little thought of what the future will bring. One supporter put it this way: 'I just take everything as it comes, everything that happens, every problem that comes up, you just take it and see what you can do, it's not that you've actually forgotten about the problems, they just come, come, come, problems keep coming up that I never knew would happen . . .'

For these reasons, it is sometimes difficult to pin down and detail the problems faced by carers of the elderly mentally infirm: the problems merge one into the other; their significance may fluctuate according to the situation of the carer, and the development of the dementia. It can be difficult to know how a problem is being defined; are all the disabilities and disturbances of the elderly dementing individual problems, and how should one interpret a supporter's report of some disability exhibited by their relative which they say is no problem?

While there have recently been a number of studies which have attempted to delineate the problems faced by supporters of the elderly mentally infirm, confusion exists in providing a conceptual separation between problems experienced as stressors and problems experienced as strain. Thus Pearlin and Schooler (1978) state 'by strain we mean those enduring problems that have the potential for arousing threat, a meaning that establishes strain and stressor as interchangeable concepts'. By so merging the concepts of strain and stressor, it becomes impossible to examine the extent to which differing problems (stressors) result in differing experiences of strain. Yet by defining problems as stressors, there is an implicit assumption that they are experienced as causing strain, difficulty or distress. The difference becomes simply one of emphasis: the stress is stimulus, the strain is the response, yet without the response, the stimulus in isolation has no significance; equally, the strain as response has meaning only in so far as it relates to a particular stimulus event, or stressor.

Even when such a separation is made, the status of a problem as a stressor (in the sense of having the potential to produce strain) is not always clear. Lazarus and DeLongis (1982) have emphasised some of the difficulties surrounding current research on stress. They point out that the dominant model in such research 'treats stress as life events that create change and require adaptation . . . [resulting in] . . . preoccupation with dramatic events and severely taxing situations'. They further note that life-events research covers a severely limited range of events, ignores the significance of non-events, and fails to recognise the extent to which certain events are probabilistically associated with life stages, and are or are not potentially anticipated by the individual.

These authors suggest that an alternative strategy is to focus on what they term 'daily hassles', which they describe as 'the irritating, frustrating, distressing demands and troubled relationships that plague people day in and day out . . . some of which are transient, others repeated or even chronic' (Lazarus and DeLongis, 1982).

Such conceptualisation of stressors as 'daily hassles' seems to better represent the situation of carers than models derived from life-events research. Nevertheless, because such problems may be continuous or chronic features of the supporters' life, they may not be mentioned spontaneously, in contrast to the more momentous events and difficulties that arise during the course of caring. Thus some studies have relied upon the spontaneous complaints of supporters describing what their main problems are, while others have presented supporters with questionnaires or checklists and asked them to identify the problems or difficulties on these self-report measures. The latter studies may select certain 'potential problems' because of their immediate concern with the cognitive–behavioural symptoms of dementia, while others may select a differing set of items based more upon the 'ageing' characteristics of the dependants. All in all, both spontaneous reports and self-report measures may provide only a selected view of the problems or stressors facing the supporters of the elderly mentally infirm. By examining differing studies, employing differing recording measures, it may nevertheless be possible to piece together the range and type of difficulties supporters face and, from such knowledge, to form the basis for developing a more individualised and comprehensive service for helping such families.

Previous Research

One of the earliest examples of research into this area is the work of Sainsbury and Grad (Sainsbury, Costain and Grad, 1965). These workers were responsible for developing and evaluating a community-based psychiatric service to the adult population of Chichester. Part of this research separately examined the situation of families caring for elderly mentally ill relatives, not all of whom were in fact suffering from dementia.

In an early report on the project, Grad and Sainsbury (1965) listed the chief problems which families reported as being sources of concern and upset in caring for their elderly dependant – namely, 'being restless and overtalkative during the day', 'being troublesome at night', 'being uncooperative and contrary', 'having hypochondriacal concerns', 'engaging in behaviour threatening others' safety', 'causing trouble with neighbours' and 'engaging in objectionable, rude or embarrassing behaviour'. It seems clear that these problems are very 'psychiatric' in nature, being a mixture of 'symptomatic behaviours' and 'psychopathology'.

A more 'geriatric' sample was investigated by Sanford (1975), the majority of the respondents being family members who were caring for a dementing relative. While also finding that night-time problems were a frequent complaint of the supporters, as was 'dangerous, irresponsible' behaviour, Sanford's group of supporters also reported problems of incontinence, falls, need for assistance in getting in and out of bed, and communication.

Clearly, these two studies illustrate an overlapping but conceptually separate group of problems facing supporters – those reflecting disability and those reflecting disturbance. The existence of separable problem dimensions can be observed in other studies which have relied upon self-report measures of problems. Both Greene *et al.* (1982) and Gilleard *et al.* (1982) used factor analysis to examine the dimensions of supporters' problem reports, though the dimensions they identified show little correspondence. The former observed three dimensions, which they labelled 'behaviour disturbance', 'apathy/withdrawal' and 'mood disturbance'; the latter reported five dimensions: 'dependency', 'disturbance', 'disability', 'demandingness' and 'wandering'. A different selection of items used in the two studies has clearly produced a lack of common problem domains.

Machin (1980), in her study of 47 supporters of elderly infirm holiday-relief hospital admissions, examined 'poorly tolerated behaviours'. These were defined as 'any problems which make life particularly difficult for the supporter'. She found incontinence, objections or refusal to being bathed or washed, nocturnal wandering and overdemanding behaviour to be most frequently cited.

However, while 31 of her supporters recorded incontinence on a behaviour-rating scale for their dependant, only seven mentioned this as a difficult problem.

When examining these studies, some common features do emerge, however; namely, that incontinence, nocturnal disturbance, demandingness, and apathy/disengagement are frequently reported to be stressful problems faced by supporters. Other studies (Isaacs, 1971; Koopman-Boyden and Wells, 1979) have shown that physical disabilities rarely are perceived as being particularly stressful aspects for caregivers, compared with mental disabilities. It seems that what is problematic is that which most distorts or disturbs the relationship between supporter and dependant. Whereas physical disabilities may be seen as signs of illness, incontinence, being woken up at night, constantly being followed about, or being asked questions, being unable (or unwilling) to engage in activities and conversations at home may all be seen as 'deliberate' attempts to inconvenience or upset the supporter, or as examples of lack of concern for the supporter. They may lead to anxieties and fears which, as well as reflecting realistic concerns, also originate from the loss of certainty, rationality and comprehensibility which serves to strain and endanger the bonds between dependant and caregiver.

To some extent, then, the problems arising from caring for the elderly mentally infirm reside in the changes in the relationship between the caregivers and their dependant, and the various disturbances and disabilities simply serve as signals of that change, which Hirschfeld (1981) has termed a loss of mutuality. Some aspects of disability are therefore less likely to be problems than others. Both Machin (1980) and Greene *et al.* (1982) found behaviours characterised by apathy and disengagement to be significantly related to the degree of strain experienced by caregivers. Likewise, Machin (1980) and Gilleard *et al.* (1982) found demanding behaviour to be associated with caregivers' reported strain. At first sight, these findings seem contradictory. However, when viewed within the context of family relationships, both sets of behaviours may be seen as reflecting an increasing ego-centredness and lack of concern on the part of the dementing person. Possibly because of the decline in the ability to integrate outside information, and with an increasingly limited field of cognitive awareness, the disinterest in conversation and shared family news and events combines with a narrow insistence on meeting needs for security (following the supporter around, repeatedly asking for help, reassurance, or simply orientation) resulting in an increasingly one-sided unrewarding relationship. One man put it like this: 'there's no sensible conversation, in the sense that she doesn't offer anything, she can't talk about anything . . . she talks continuously, a loud whisper, always wanting to go home, wanting to go home, continually talking about her mother "I want to see my mother", and wanting to go home.' The inability to give anything to the relationship and the impossible nature of the demands produce a lack of reciprocity which is most acutely felt by those who have lived interdependent lives for a considerable length of time. Often, too, this inability to share causes both frustration and guilt, the latter arising from a feeling that underneath their partner or parent is really trying to communicate, but they can no longer decipher the message. Another supporter said 'there's something in her mind still working, still troubling her that she's like this, but she can't say what it is'.

Barnes *et al.* (1981), in discussing the problems surrounding the development of dementia, have drawn attention to the difficulties associated with the lack of affectional and indeed sexual responsivity of dementing spouses, and the resulting loss of emotional sustenance experienced by their partners. At the same time, because of fears of embarrassment and because of the need for continual supervision, social isolation of the supporter increasingly meant that such supporters failed to gain social and emotional sustenance from relationships outside the home.

The Edinburgh Research Studies

Because of the need to assess behavioural disabilities and disturbances separately from their status as problems, we have tried in our own research to develop a measure which may reflect more sensitively the prevalence of differing potential stressors facing caregivers. Originally, we developed a problem checklist, from which supporters of mentally infirm day-hospital attenders were asked to identify problems they were currently facing (Gilleard and Watt, 1982). Then, recognising the distinction made by many supporters between noticing their dependants' disabilities and labelling them as problems, we revised the format to include separate ratings of occurrence of deficit or disturbing behaviours, and their 'problem' status for the supporter. At this stage, we also expanded the range of potential problems by including additional items, particularly those reflecting inactivity and disengagement, which Greene *et al.* (1982) had identified as particularly stressful. We also tried, and then later abandoned, an attempt to include what Sanford (1975) had termed 'alleviation' factors – asking the supporters which problems would need to be alleviated to make the situation more tolerable. Our reason for not pursuing this strategy was that for a considerable number of supporters there was no desire to give up caring for their dependant, while for others the issue was not one of a specific set of problems requiring alleviation, but rather that a whole complex of behavioural disabilities and disturbances surround them, from which it was not possible to identify individual problems which would, if altered, remedy the situation.

Thus we felt it pointless to insist on seeking a metric of problem tolerance, and concentrated our efforts on devising a comprehensive recording of deficits, disturbances and disabilities, together with their subjectively perceived severity. This final version of the problem checklist is reproduced at the end of the book, as an appendix.

Much of the information described in the rest of this chapter is based upon research into groups of supporters whose dependant was referred for, or attended psychogeriatric or geriatric day-hospital care. The fact that both the dementing people and the supporters are still living and facing the difficulties of dementia in the community, that such attenders demonstrate considerable variation in severity of dementia, and that the identification of such families and the principal supporter is relatively easy made this group in many ways ideal to yield information on the problems facing caregivers of the elderly mentally infirm. We cannot, of course, be sure how representative such groups are of all those who are in the position of caring for the elderly mentally infirm, but most, if not all, were prepared to continue caring for their dependant at home, at least for the time being.

Three main studies have been completed, the first made up from 53 supporters with a dependant attending one of three day hospitals in the City of Edinburgh, the second from a series of 129 consecutive referrals to psychogeriatric day-hospital care in the Lothian region, and the third a random sample ($n = 205$) of supporters of day-hospital attenders drawn from all day hospitals (geriatric and psychogeriatric) in Scotland. This latter group consisted of 119 supporters of a mentally impaired day patient, and 88 supporters of a mentally unimpaired day patient.

Table 5.1: Occurrence of Problems Presented to the Supporters by their Elderly Mentally Infirm Dependants

Problem	Study 1 $n = 53$	Study 2 $n = 129$	Study 3 EPI $n = 119$	EMI $n = 85$	
1. Not safe outside alone	83	79	94	77	*
2. Unsteady on feet	85	77	87	96	
3. Disrupts personal/social life	79	66	87	70	*
4. Forgets things that have happened	75	95	94 96	74	***
5. Unable to dress without help	74	56	86	73	
6. Unable to hold a sensible conversation	68	74	81	37	***
7. Always asking questions	68	58	64	48	**
8. Demands attention	66	66	84	72	
9. Careless about own appearance	58	61	55	27	***
10. Temper outbursts	47	59	65	34	***
11. Cannot be left alone for even one hour	55	50	67	51	***
12. Unable to wash without help	55	58	81	71	
13. Falling	55	51	66	61	
14. No concern for personal hygiene	51	53	48	25	***
15. Unable to walk outside the house	51	38	69	76	
16. Unable to manage stairs	49	49	65	84	**
17. Wanders about the house at night	47	55	52	10	***
18. Creates personality clashes	45	51	50	33	*
19. Physically too heavy to move easily	43	(38%)	63	78	
20. Incontinent (soiling)	40	36	61	43	*
21. Incontinent (wetting)	38	34	55	56	
22. Physically aggressive	32	32	27	10	*
23. Needs help at mealtimes	30	27	60	54	
24. Unable to get in or out of bed without help	25	32	61	75	
25. Vulgar habits	23	23	28	6	***
26. Noisy, shouts	21	31	29	16	
27. Bad language	17	25	31	15	*
28. Rude to visitors	13	23	24	6	**
29. Unable to take part in family conversation	—	67	79	44	***
30. Unable to read newspapers and magazines	—	81	74	54	**
31. Sits around doing nothing	—	97	98	84	**
32. No interest in news of friends or family	—	78	61	24	***
33. Unable to follow TV (or radio)	—	75	71	36	***
34. Unable to occupy self doing useful things	—	85	95	70	***

Notes: 1. A significant difference in occurrence of the problem between mentally deteriorated and mentally normal dependants was tested by χ^2; the probability of significant differences are indicated thus:
  * P < 0.05, ** P < 0.01, *** P < 0.001
2. Numbers in columns refer to percentages.
3. EPI = elderly physically infirm; EMI = elderly mentally infirm.

The first item of information we sought was to identify how frequent various behavioural disturbances and disabilities were in our groups. Though each item on the checklist is coded for frequency of occurrence, we have initially focused upon which features are present, irrespective of frequency. The information is supplied in Table 5.1

When compared with our earlier work (Gilleard and Watt, 1982) relying upon spontaneous indications of 'problems', it has been apparent that, as currently used, the checklist produces a much greater frequency of reporting of disabilities, as Machin's (1980) study indicated to be the case with reports of incontinence. The existence of a disability is not the same as the existence of a problem, in the supporters' eyes. While 29 per cent reported temper outbursts as a problem in our original survey, in the present samples, frequency of occurrence is almost 60 per cent. Further evidence of the importance of this distinction has recently been found by Eagles (1983). Using an earlier 28-item version of the problem checklist, he compared hospital staff's and supporters' reports of problems presented by a series of new admissions to a psychogeriatric unit, who were suffering from dementia. His results demonstrated a comparative 'under-reporting' of problems by relatives, which was most marked in those relatives who subsequently took their dependant back home, on discharge. The objective recording of disabilities may be much less important, and is certainly not the same as the subjective reporting of problems by supporters.

However, what Table 5.1 does indicate is the frequency with which certain disabilities occur in dementing people living in the community. Nearly all supporters feel that their relative is not safe outside on their own, they spend a lot of time sitting around at home doing nothing, they cannot occupy themselves, they seem unsteady on their feet, and naturally forget things that have just happened. The majority of supporters also describe their relative as unable to maintain a sensible conversation, or to take part in family conversation, they show no interest in family news, and need help in such self-care activities as dressing and washing. Constant questioning and demands for attention, disruption of personal social life and lack of concern for their appearance and personal hygiene also are reported in the majority of cases, as is a proneness to falls.

Incontinence, mobility problems and rude or aggressive behaviour characterise a sizeable minority of the dependants, though the latter are relatively infrequently reported compared with the problems of dependency, demandingness and particularly disinterest and apathy.

When those with mental infirmity are contrasted with those dependants whose primary infirmity is physical rather than mental, in study 3, what is most apparent is that the difference lies mainly in the absence of apathy, demandingness, indifference to self-care and behaviour disturbance in the latter group, rather than any absence of mobility or self-care impairment among the mentally infirm. For the majority of supporters of the elderly mentally infirm attending day hospitals, the difficulties of physical dependency are compounded by additional, rather than different, handicaps of a cognitive, motivational and social nature.

Table 5.2 examines the 'problems' reported by the supporters. As stated earlier, there are good reasons to consider separately reports of disabilities from reports of problems. While a problem reflects a disability, a disability does not necessitate the existence of a problem; thus several disability items are rated as presenting 'no problem' to the supporter.

No disability or disturbed behaviour is perceived as 'a problem' by all the supporters, although item 11 'cannot be left on their own for even one hour' comes nearest to being universally described as a problem by the supporters. Considering first the 'major problems', the data in Table 5.2 suggest that the need for supervision, in and out of the house, proneness to falls, incontinence, night-time wandering and the inability to occupy him or herself present the greatest difficulties to supporters. One may assume that the supporters who perceive their dependant to be unsafe and at risk, and who consequently feel the need for constant supervision, are those experiencing the greatest problems, and are most likely to feel themselves under strain. Also, a frequently problematic aspect of behaviour is the inability of the dependant to show interest in conversations or indeed to do anything to occupy themselves (items 6, 29 and 34). It can be argued that such disinterest and apathy provide a frustrating sense of needing to do something for the person, and also that the supporters cannot, on the whole, ignore and leave their dependant unresponsive and inactive without considerable upset to themselves.

Surprisingly, problems of aggression, abuse and hostility (items 10, 22, 26, 27 and 28) are seen as great problems by less than a quarter of the supporters who describe the occurrence of such

Table 5.2: Severity of Problem Ratings of Disabilities and Disturbances Reported by Supporters of the Elderly Mentally Infirm

Problem		Study 2			Study 3 (EMI group)		
		No problem	Some	Great problem	No problem	Some	Great problem
1. Not safe outside alone	277	15	30	55	13	39	49
2. Unsteady on feet	259	14	47	38	10	44	46
3. Disrupts personal and social life	263	20	38	42	7	45	48
4. Forgets things that have happened	231	23	39	38	21	42	37
5. Unable to dress without help	185	29	47	24	31	48	21
6. Unable to hold a sensible conversation	260	17	45	38	11	39	50
7. Always asking questions	195	22	53	26	37	36	27
8. Demands attention	241	17	41	42	17	50	33
9. Careless about own appearance	143	32	39	29	24	53	22
10. Temper outbursts	209	17	58	25	20	59	21
11. Cannot be left alone for even one hour	335	4	25	71	0	32	68
12. Unable to wash without help	194	26	48	26	27	52	21
13. Falling	260	14	46	40	8	50	42
14. No concern for personal hygiene	247	24	28	48	10	57	33
15. Unable to walk outside the home	233	24	41	35	18	42	40
16. Unable to manage stairs	180	43	38	19	21	54	25
17. Wanders about the house at night	280	16	42	42	6	34	60
18. Creates personality clashes	228	18	54	28	16	50	34
19. Unable to get out of a chair without help	184	47	27	27	24	49	27
20. Incontinent (soiling)	246	14	38	48	23	42	35
21. Incontinent (wetting)	252	23	29	49	14	45	40
22. Physically aggressive	220	13	53	33	21	59	21
23. Needs help at meals	146	40	44	16	39	52	9
24. Unable to get in and out of bed without help	176	47	27	26	27	49	24
25. Vulgar habits	224	16	55	29	14	61	25
26. Noisy, shouts	185	34	42	24	22	63	16
27. Bad language	179	35	42	23	32	48	19
28. Rude to visitors	181	43	44	13	11	67	22
29. Unable to take part in family conversations	235	30	35	35	18	34	48
30. Unable to read newspapers and magazines	176	33	38	29	40	40	20
31. Sits around doing nothing	208	31	28	41	34	34	32
32. No interest in news of friends and family	160	35	48	17	37	48	15
33. Unable to follow TV (or radio)	161	43	35	22	35	48	17
34. Unable to occupy self doing useful things	239	27	23	50	24	36	40

Note: Numbers in columns refer to percentages.

behaviours. Perhaps because those behaviours are 'occasional' rather than 'constant', they may be less significant sources of strain than the ever-present need for supervision, and lack of responsivity which characterise problems of 'not being able to be left alone', 'sitting around doing nothing' and 'not being able to hold a sensible conversation'.

Clearly, the implications of these findings have relevance for the kind of services most likely to benefit supporters. In the first place must come relief from constant supervision, a role which psychogeriatric day hospitals, day centres and even the home-help service may serve. Secondly, the lack of activity which obviously distresses supporters may also be met, to some extent, by day-care services. Perhaps the most frequent benefit of psychogeriatric day care reported by supporters, after its role of providing time out, is that it is a place where their dependant can meet people, and 'do things'. What they do and whether they remember what they have done may be less important than the belief that they are being kept active and engaged, a task for which the supporter may feel they no longer have the resources. It can be argued that the failure to act and to react represents a failure to be a person, and this lack of identity will most threaten the sense of mutuality which seems necessary to sustain the caring relationship. Thirdly, specific 'symptomatic behaviours', such as incontinence and nocturnal wandering are a major problem – though not, it would appear, hostility or abusiveness. The practical resources of an incontinent laundry service, commodes for loan, and district and night nursing services for dependants too heavy to lift, toilet and change are some obvious service provisions, currently irregularly available, which seem appropriate. Night-time wandering, a frequently noted stressor for the supporters, is obviously open to pharmacological intervention, though night sedation frequently results in drowsiness and cognitive and motor impairments the next day. Some recent evidence, however, does suggest that short half-life hypnotics (i.e. sedatives which are rapidly eliminated from tissue) may not have so great adverse day-time effects, even with the elderly mentally infirm (Mead and Castleden, 1982). Alternatively, manipulation of the physical environment and the reduction of day-time inactivity may also be recommendations that community occupational therapists or health visitors could facilitate. Some supporters hit on such solutions themselves. One husband removed the bathroom door, installed a night light, and placed cushioning along the skirting boards to minimise, to his satisfaction, the effects of his wife's habit of wandering about at night. Sometimes more drastic measures are taken. Two sisters who were looking after their dementing sister had to sleep on either side of her to prevent her getting up and wandering off at night. Successful prevention often meant that they got up in the morning black and blue from bruises as a result of their efforts.

Fourthly, while major immobility (items 16, 19 and 24) is often not a great problem, unsteadiness and proneness to falls (items 2 and 13) clearly are. If, as seems likely, these problems present difficulties because the mentally impaired cannot be relied upon to take account of their own infirmities, it is important that the risks of serious falls are minimised. Again, community occupational therapists, and perhaps health visitors or social workers, may be in a position to advise supporters on how to spot potential hazards in the home, to make recommendations regarding suitable footwear and to assist supporters in obtaining aids such as handrails, non-slip bath mats, etc. and replace steps with ramps and so forth.

Finally, it must be recognised that aside from specific sets of problems described by supporters caring for a dementing person in the community, more diffuse problems exist – the restrictions on personal social life and the resentment this causes, the sadness at witnessing the deterioration of mind and manners in a parent or partner. Barnes *et al.* (1981) have described how many supporters experience 'the difficulty of grieving for the loss of their "dead" companion who was still physically present but slowly deteriorating', and the resulting wishes and fantasies for their dependant's early death.

Summary

The problems arising from caring for a dementing relative are not fixed, but represent a dynamic pattern of development. In the early stages, problems focus upon identification and the uncertainty generated by the feeling that all is not well with the relative, but without the supporter necessarily knowing what is wrong, or why. Social and emotional withdrawal and apathy prove increasingly problematic, as they alter and reduce the reciprocity that had existed between supporter and dependant.

At the same time, fears for the safety of the dependant and an increasing awareness of the need to supervise their actions place increasing demands upon the supporter, who may be further stressed by the attention-seeking and security-seeking which leads their dependant to follow them around, repeatedly ask questions and seek reassurance.

Finally, growing deterioration in personal habits (incontinence, no concern for hygiene) seems to further alienate and cause problems for the supporter, probably because such deterioration makes the dependant even less like the person who was once known and loved.

Night-time disturbance and the disruptive effects of a 24-hour need for supervision, when even at night the person remains at risk for behaving inappropriately or dangerously, compound the difficulties. As some recent authors have put it, such developing problems lead many supporters to be living 'The 36-Hour Day' (Mace and Robins, 1981).

6 LIVING WITH DEMENTIA: THE CONSEQUENCES OF CARING

Issues of Measurement

While several researchers have indicated the problems that face the supporters of the elderly mentally infirm, others have emphasised more the psychosocial consequences of having to deal with such problems. In the previous chapter, attention was drawn to the overlapping concepts of stressor and strain, and the difficulties of focusing purely on the responses to situations, life-events or hassles, as though the former are located inside the person, while the latter exist 'out there', in the social and physical environment. Nevertheless it is helpful to make such a separation, if only to permit a different emphasis and bring out different links existing between stress and strain. Thus, in this chapter the emphasis is less upon what problems the behaviour of the dementing person presents to the supporter, but rather what reactions and responses are evinced by these problems within the supporter and what factors mediate the experience of strain.

That caring for a family member or friend who is dementing can be enormously stressful has long been recognised, by both clinicians (e.g. Sheldon, 1948; Macmillan, 1960, 1967) and researchers (Grad and Sainsbury, 1965). More recently, however, research interest has been devoted to providing quantitative indices of strain, which can then be used to examine variations within groups of supporters, to identify mitigating or exacerbating influences on the response of caregivers, to compare the relative strain associated with different types and degrees of infirmity in those being cared for, and of course to evaluate the impact of service aid on reducing such strain. Clearly, it is desirable for these and other reasons to progress from simply emphasising that such caregiving is a source of strain, to quantifying and determining how much of a strain, for which supporters, under what circumstances.

The work of Grad and Sainsbury (1965) represents some of the earliest attempts to provide such quantification. They developed an overall rating of family burden, based upon separate ratings of (i) strain on the mental health of families caring for an elderly mentally ill relative, (ii) strain on their social life, (iii) strain on their physical health, and (iv) strain on their financial resources. Each of these four areas of strain or burden were rated as 'no burden', 'some burden' and 'severe burden', and the global rating was similarly trichotomised. These ratings were made by social workers based upon interviews with family members. Their findings indicated the marked prevalence of burden (40 per cent given 'severe' burden ratings, 40 per cent 'some burden'), which was most marked in the areas of social life, and mental health; only 3 per cent of the families interviewed were under severe burden for their physical health and 6 per cent for their financial well-being. Such findings have generally been endorsed by many other subsequent researchers (Fengler and Goodrich, 1979; Archbold, 1981), namely, that the primary expression of strain is in psychosocial impairment, rather than in physical or financial well-being.

While Grad and Sainsbury (1965) used a restricted three-point scale, they clearly recognised the multidimensional nature of burden or strain. Many subsequent studies that have employed quantitative indices have, however, concentrated upon developing single indices of strain (Machin, 1980; Zarit, Reever and Bach-Peterson, 1980; Robinson, 1983). Greene *et al.* (1982) subjected their own strain scale to a factor analysis, and observed a three-dimensional solution, encompassing domestic upset, personal distress and supporters' negativity towards their dependant. Other researchers have concentrated on measures of morale, rather than strain or burden (e.g. Fengler and Goodrich, 1979; Gilhooley, 1984a), which are less direct indices of strain and burden. One approach has been to employ measures of emotional distress, such as symptom checklists (Zarit *et al.*, 1980), or global ratings of mental health (Gilhooley, 1984a), in addition to indices of strain or burden. Still others have derived arbitrary indices of negative consequences or strain based upon open-ended interview questions (Hirschfield, 1981; Johnson and Catalona, 1982).

Clearly, the measurement of strain is an unresolved area for research, and as long as this situation persists, there needs to be considerable caution in linking findings from differing studies, both with respect to the extent of strain and the factors associated with observed variations in strain amongst supporting relatives. Is low morale to be considered equivalent to severe strain, or marked depression, or severe burden? A conceptually adequate index requires not simply an agreed measure of strain, but an adequate conceptualisation of what aspects of the negative consequences of caregiving are being examined. For example, it is one thing to say 'I am under strain', another to say 'looking after Dad is a great strain'. The former, like morale, is a situationally independent statement of negative feeling, the latter, like burden, is a subjective judgement of the felt negativity of a situation. Thus one may feel that looking after someone is quite a burden, and yet feel that one remains essentially in good spirits (high morale, low distress). A further distinction can be made between measures focusing upon the feelings of the supporter and those focusing on the restrictions in life-style imposed on the supporter in connection with their caregiving activities.

caregiving different depending on the disease?

Current Research Findings on Factors Influencing Strain

Horowitz (1981, 1982a) produced a 'caregiving-consequences scale', based upon interview data concerned with changes occurring in supporters' life-styles as a result of their caregiving. While her sample focused upon the 'infirm' elderly, only a proportion of the dependants were significantly mentally impaired. Nevertheless, there were highly significant correlations between degree of memory impairment, degree of impairment in self-care skills, and the summed total of the 'caregiving-consequences' scale, suggesting that caring for the mentally impaired creates significantly more negative impact on supporters than caring for the mentally unimpaired infirm elderly. Similar findings were obtained in the study by Klusmann *et al.* (1981), who found that relatives taking care of physically relatively healthy parents with moderate-to-severe dementia reported the greatest strain (low morale, high number of psychosomatic complaints) especially compared with those taking care of severely physically infirm parents.

Surprisingly, Zarit *et al.* (1980) found no such correlations between reported feelings of burden amongst supporters and the number of memory and behaviour impairments of their mentally impaired dependant. This finding was subsequently replicated in a later study (Zarit, Gatz and Zarit, 1981), for both their index of burden and an index of emotional distress, based on common psychiatric symptom complaints. While Horowitz's sample included both mentally unimpaired as well as mentally impaired elderly, Zarit's group was made up only of spouses of elderly dementia patients. Thus it may be that while the presence of demen-

LIT REVIEW ꜱᴛ (RECENT)
ON CAREGIVING FOR ELDERLY
WITH
DEMENTIA.

tia is itself a significant factor in determining strain or burden in caregiving, differing degrees of dementia are not so closely associated with differing degrees of strain.

Given the different types of measures used to assess strain, and the consequent caution required in interpreting findings from different studies, what factors seem to play a part in producing strain? Both the Horowitz and the Zarit studies have approached this problem by using multiple regression analysis – a multivariate statistical technique which enables the investigator to assess the unique contribution of several variables to predicting variation in the independent variable, in this case burden or 'negative consequences'.

Zarit *et al.* (1981) found that 'social supports are more important predictors of burden than actual impairments or changes in their role in the family', such that lower levels of reported social support produced a greater sense of burden and distress. In a later expanded report of the study, Zarit (1982) noted significant sex differences in the associations between burden, support and problems. She found that husbands of dementing wives showed a straightforward relationship between the frequency and use of social supports and decreased feelings of burden, while this relationship was almost inverted for wives of dementing husbands. Thus having help outside the home (day care) and having paid help in the home were both associated with wives' reporting increased burden. Zarit speculated that this was because of differential sex-role expectations in relation to caring; wives either felt guilty about not being able to provide the care themselves, or were not able to rid themselves of the emotional burden, even when their dementing husband was away, or when they left their husband at home, under care, to get out. Thus more wives felt the problems never left them, despite physical separations. Husbands, on the other hand, felt more able to leave 'housekeeping' and 'care/supervision' to external service providers, with little emotional constraints or guilt.

ie) wives
& family
months.
is/y of
caring,
or b ut
diff dep.
on the
disease?

These interesting sex differences in burden and its correlates are clearly deserving of further investigation, for they have obvious implications in counselling family members looking after a dementing relative. Horowitz (1981) has found similar sex differences in adult children supporters, observing that daughters, unlike sons, engage in more direct 'hands-on' caregiving activities, make less use of added support from their family, have differing expectations of their own spouse with regards parent caring, and appear to be more vulnerable to strain and distress, quite independently of the level of care they have to give.

Horowitz again makes the point about gender-appropriate care-giving expectations, noting that since males do not, in general, help more in their own households even when their wives work, there is little reason to expect them to change their behaviour in relation to their own parents. Further, she points out that, although sons expect active support from their spouses while giving care to their own parent, daughters' expectations are more that their husband remains neutral and does not voice objections to their own care-giving activities, rather than that they should expect concrete help. Even so, when matched for the level of involvement in caregiving, Horowitz still found that daughters reported relatively greater strain than sons. Perhaps, as Zarit found with spouses, the involvement of daughters is more global and less confined to contact time, compared with sons, so that they continue to worry about their parent even when not with them.

Aside from these indicative sex differences, Horowitz also observes a relationship between strain and two other important variables – services and felt affection. For her adult children sup-porters, strain was significantly related to the expressed satisfaction or dissatisfaction with the current level of service provision to their infirm parent – the less satisfaction being associated with greater reported strain. Absolute level of formal support was unrelated to strain. Such a finding, she argues, indicates that it is the mismatch between level of provision and level of supporters' need that is crucial, not the absolute level of services provided. Of course, direction of causality is open to interpretation; it could equally be the case that experienced strain enhances the need for extra services.

Gilhooley (1984a), concentrating, like Zarit, on supporters of the mentally impaired elderly, also examined the correlates of well-being and strain. Like all other investigators, she found that males had higher morale, which she ascribed to their lower level of emotional involvement and their willingness to leave their depen-dant unattended. Obviously, these two are related phenomena and, given the high problem-rating ascribed to being unable to leave one's dependant alone, noted in the previous chapter, this willing-ness to leave their dependant alone may well give a degree of protection to males, which female supporters do not manage to gain. Such female overprotectiveness (or male underprotective-ness) may itself be the consequence of earlier caring experience, notably with young children. Gilhooley also found no association between level of impairment, amount of family help received and morale; like Horowitz, however, she did find that satisfaction with help received from the family correlated positively, but, as was pointed out, this gives rise to questions of causality. Of particular interest in this study is the association between formal services received and morale. She found that visits from community (district) nurses and home helps were positively associated with higher morale. Finally, morale of supporters caring for a female dependant was higher than those caring for a male dependant. This latter finding will be discussed in more detail later.

Clearly, the relationship between services received and supporters' morale or strain is an important issue, but one as yet unresolved, primarily because of the cross-sectional nature of the studies reported. If formal support is reactive to supporter strain, then, as Zarit found in her sample of wives, a positive correlation may emerge: if, on the other hand, formal support is preventive of strain, then findings such as those by Gilhooley might be expected. A mixture of reactivity and compensatory influences may result in no overall association, as Horowitz found. In order to judge more clearly the influence of formal support services on the caregiving supporter, a longitudinal intervention study is required that could help answer such questions as how helpful are day care, home helps, district nurse visiting and so on. At present, there is no clear evidence to answer these questions from existing research.

Finally, some studies have examined the question of affectional bonds between supporter and dependant, as a factor mediating the experienced burden or strain in caregiving to the elderly mentally infirm. This issue has been investigated by Horowitz and Shindelman (1981) and Hirschfeld (1981), and less directly by Gilhooley (1984a) and Klusmann *et al.* (1981).

Hirschfeld (1981) developed the concept of mutuality as 'the crucial variable determining a family's ability to continue caring for a senile brain diseased person in the home'. She defined mutuality as 'the caregiver's ability to find gratification in the relationship with the impaired person and meaning from the caregiving situation'. She also makes the important point that mutuality may be either internally reinforced, where value is determined by the supporters' own perceptions of their role and the meaning of caregiving, or externally reinforced, whereby the person being cared for provides rewards and gives meaning to their supporters' caregiving. In

Klusmann's study, the research team found that their 'intimacy' scale revealed a reduced degree of closeness in those supporters caring for a severely demented dependant, which was especially the case when the dependant was physically reasonably healthy; but when 'closeness' was rated by an observer, rather than the relative, no such relationship existed (Klusmann *et al.*, 1981). An obvious problem is posed by this study, namely, how best to define or determine closeness or mutuality and how to interpret self-reported versus observer-rated measures. Hirschfeld clearly amalgamates the external and internal reinforcements within her concept of mutuality, which she derives from open-ended questioning (for example, how much of a loss would it be if their dependant died or was institutionalised?). Such items are also incorporated in Klusmann's intimacy scale. It would seem that the ability to derive mutuality is reduced by the caregiving experience involved in looking after a dementing relative, but those supporters who can maintain such closeness seem particularly prepared to continue to care, although Hirschfeld does not state at what cost, in terms of the caregivers' morale.

A more explicit association between closeness/affection and reduced strain has been drawn by Horowitz and Shindelman. They developed from a structured interview a scale of felt affection, made up of feelings of love and closeness, in the past and in the present, and the extent to which current caregiving was motivated by explicitly affectional attitudes. She found that higher 'affection' scores were associated with less reported strain. On the other hand, a measure of 'reciprocity', credits earned from the past by the dependant, was unrelated to strain, but positively associated with the extent of involvement in caregiving. Gilhooley (1984a), using a global observer rating of quality of past relationship, found no such association with supporters' morale in her study.

Clearly, the role of past and present emotional bonds is an important one, but, like that of support, is one which is in need of further investigation. Concepts of mutuality, affection, closeness and reciprocity are interlinked, but seem to entail differing elements in the supporter – dependant relationship. One dimension requiring elucidation is that of present versus past feelings of closeness, while the second is that of bonds of duty or credits due versus emotional attachment. A close and loving relationship in the past may make adjustment considerably more difficult if the current relationship is soured by the breakdown of current mutuality resulting from dementia. On the other hand, a sense of duty and commitment may result in a willingness to care, but it may provide very little protection from the strains arising from a lack of any experienced sharing between supporter and dependant. Occasionally, a poor relationship in the past may act as a spur to caring. One middle-aged daughter visited and looked after her dementing mother, driven by a desire to at last extract some love and appreciation of which she had felt deprived throughout her childhood and young adulthood. Her involvement did little to reduce the strains imposed, but resulted in an extreme reluctance to give up on her mother.

Many motives and many strategies can thus be observed amongst supporters in their attempts to cope with the task of giving care to their dementing relative. The next section will consider what role such coping strategies play in influencing the strains of caregiving.

Caring, Coping and Managing Strategies: Their Influence on Strain

Several researchers have examined the methods of coping or managing employed by supporters looking after an elderly infirm relative. Some have focused upon the general style of management, whereas others have examined in more detail the range and variety of coping strategies employed. Finally, a few have examined differences in levels of strain or morale in relation to these different strategies.

A detailed analysis of what caregivers do when looking after an elderly mentally infirm relative is lacking. Horowitz (1981) has listed ten areas of caregiving involvement, ranging from health and personal care to financial assistance and management, but these are very broad areas of 'services' which omit the role of supervision, prevention of accidents, acts of constant reassurance, persuasion to take medication and so forth that make up the round of daily hassles in caretaking for many supporters. One husband would take his wife shopping, and, in so doing, developed a series of routes which would reduce the distance from public lavatories with attendants on hand to help his wife. Another woman went to considerable trouble to arrange a volunteer visitor for her mildly dementing husband who could sit and play a game of chess with him. Such acts involve shielding and reducing environmental pressures which might threaten the behavioural competence of the dementing person, enhancing what Lawton has described as the ecological fit between person and environment (Lawton and Nahemow, 1973).

Many successful strategies indicate the potential resourcefulness of relatives in assisting the personal survival of their dependant, and these could potentially be brought together into a comprehensive manual of a 'what to do if he/she . . .' nature. At present, this resource is lacking in its entirety, though the necessary elements of ingenuity and adaptiveness will be found in many supporters' care-giving stories. Gilhooley (1980) has called these 'behavioural' coping strategies, in contrast to 'psychological' coping strategies; the latter reflect more a coping perspective or set of attitudes that may help maintain caregivers' morale, or reduce the strain they face.

At a much broader level, Archbold (1981) has analysed the caregiving strategies of women caring for chronically ill, severely functionally impaired parents, categorising caregiving into two roles: care-managing and care-providing. She identifies these patterns as follows: 'the care manager identifies the needed services and manages their provision by others; the care provider identifies the services needed and performs them herself'. In her American study, she found that care managers came from higher socio-economic backgrounds, they were more likely to be employed full-time in socially valued careers, whose importance, Archbold felt, reduced the scope for conflict between parent care-providing and work. Characteristic also of such care managers was a social network that included physicians, lawyers, social workers and nurses. Care providers, on the other hand, were poorer, had limited social networks and, if employed, had low-status jobs; naturally, care providers were found to be under greater strain and found considerably less satisfaction in their caregiving role than did the care managers.

While the adult child is capable of occupying one of Archbold's general management positions, spouses are not often in a position to act as care managers. Almost inevitably they will be care providers. Zarit's (1982) study suggests that husbands may be able to adopt more effective coping strategies than women, simply because they can opt out of, or at least reduce, many of the needed domestic and personal care chores by relying upon traditional sex-role models of caring. Thus community services (home helps, district nurses) and the informal services of adult children (daughters, daughters-in-law), provided by women, can be easily accepted, and care-providing responsibilities minimised without censure by such husbands.

Gilhooley (1980) found in her sample of supporters that men more often than women, employed such behavioural coping strategies and coincidentally reported higher morale. She also described coping strategies that involved minimising problems or ignoring the dependant which were also associated with supporters' maintained morale. Such distancing or disengaging strategies may operate at a behavioural or at an interpersonal level, however. An example of the latter can be illustrated by the following case: a middle-aged daughter, married, with teenage children, visited her dementing mother's house on the way to work, at lunchtime and in the evening, every day. She would get her mother up, prepare breakfast, ensuring that some was eaten, and light the fire. At lunchtime she would briefly tidy the house, make the bed (or get her mother out of bed if she had returned there), and make lunch – usually soup and sandwiches. She would take home dirty clothes to be washed at her own home. In the evening, she would call round to ensure her mother was all right and return home. During this time her communication with her mother was primarily functional, even authoritarian. When I visited, she sat her mother down on the settee and proceeded to discuss her disabilities calmly and in matter-of-fact terms, with little recognition of any possible upset this may have caused her mother. As far as she was concerned her mother could no longer grasp conversations, so it did not matter. In some sense she felt her mother had died, and her caregiving involvement reflected a historical duty to what her mother had been. While her behaviour reflected the recognition of the physical and security needs of her mother, emotionally she no longer recognised any continuing interpersonal duty. Such depersonalised care may easily be criticised, but it clearly served an adaptive function which had effectively reduced the distress that had originally been experienced during the early stages of her mother's deterioration.

Johnson and Catelona (1982) have identified such distancing strategies in the adult children of infirm elderly parents discharged from hospital. They found that there were important differences, however, in the coping strategies employed by children and spouses. They distinguished between two broadly opposing styles of adaptation in caregivers – distancing and enmeshing techniques, the former being primarily employed by children, the latter primarily by spouses. Distancing may involve a physical distancing, when the caregiver ceases to visit or arranges the transfer of caregiving responsibility to others, including of course institutions. An example of such physical distancing can be illustrated by another case investigated by the author. This woman had experienced considerable upset in her visits to her mildly dementing, rather paranoid mother. She had failed to enlist for her mother much in the way of community services, and was regularly abused by her mother for not doing things right, for not getting the right shopping, for making a mess of the living room and so on. Frequently her mother would refuse to eat the meals she prepared – mother and daughter lived close to each other. The daughter reduced her visits over the next six months until she virtually saw her mother only once or twice a fortnight, though her husband, with whom the mother got on well, continued daily visits to keep an eye on things, make the fire and collect laundry. A home help had begun visiting. As Johnson and Catelona noted, such a response usually reflects considerable anger and resentment over the parents' disabilities. It is interesting to note, in Isaacs *et al.*'s (1972) study of supporters of elderly geriatric admission patients, that the minority of children these authors found not to be supporting a lone elderly parent tended to have maintained their physical distance for similar reasons of hostility and anger over their parents' behaviour, often reflecting lifelong patterns of resentment at their unacceptable personality traits.

The second form of distancing Johnson and Catelona term 'establishing psychological distance while maintaining physical proximity'. This strategy involves ignoring the problems and emotional demands of the dependant to the extent of 'avoiding all interactions other than those which provide instrumental supports' (Johnson and Catalona, 1982), similar to the 'ignoring' described by Gilhooley (1980) and illustrated above in the case of the visiting daughter.

A third form of distancing is also described – what may be termed a diffusion of responsibility. This involves a strategy similar to Archbold's care-managing approach, whereby the caregiver (again, usually an adult child) involves other family members and enlists formal supports to share out the caregiving. Such a strategy is obviously dependent upon a reasonably integrated family structure, with other siblings and relatives living close at hand and accepting the responsibilities of such additional caregiving. Occasionally, this strategy can be observed amongst siblings, where one sister moves in to share the household of a second, who has been looking after the third, dependent sister. In such cases, a common bond of widowhood and the material advantages of sharing a common household may compensate for the undesirable difficulties of dealing with the dementing sibling's needs. Jerrome (1981) has pointed out how, in late life, the desire to maintain social networks and friendships can often lead to an intensification of relationships between siblings and indeed cousins, who may have been quite distant or even unfriendly in earlier years. Such development of latent kin relationships may be a great advantage to those from large families, an option that will become increasingly less available to future generations of 'two children' families.

In contrast to distancing and diffusion of responsibility, Johnson and Catalona describe supporting relatives who employ 'enmeshing' techniques which serve to draw caregiver and dependant into a closer, more interdependent relationship. They further describe two particular enmeshing techniques, which they term 'social regression' and 'role entrenchment', both of which may be evident particularly amongst spouse caregivers. Social regression refers to the increasing isolation from other relationships and involvements which the caregiver gives up to devote the majority of his or her time to the caregiving tasks. The extent to which such imposed isolation is forced upon a spouse through lack of alternative family and other informal supports, and the extent to which it is self-selected is often difficult to establish. In some ways, this strategy merges into that of role entrenchment, which these authors define as 'a situation in which the caregiver redefines his or her role by enlarging its content and reconceptualising the costs and benefits accruing from the arrangement'. In other words, when circumstances force the healthier partner to cut off or reduce external social relationships, they may cope by rationalising their exclusive caregiving role to take on the attributes of a new purpose in life. The extent to which this new investment in caring may become so valuable, despite the objective stresses involved, can be observed in some spouses of patients referred for psychogeriatric day care. On the days when they are released from caring, they may find themselves uncomfortably at a loss for what to do, how to spend their time, as though without the daily round of caregiving they could only confront the absence of any other goals in their life. Such individuals may worry how their partner is getting on at the day hospital, and feel that perhaps the staff do not really understand their needs and appreciate their habits. Providing care and adapting to each new problem posed by their dementing partner becomes a means of maintaining self-esteem; it is necessary therefore to believe that others cannot fully compete in caregiving skill and competence. Providing staff accept and do not challenge such beliefs, day care can be tolerated and the caregiver can often re-establish social contacts and interests that had been given up. Occasionally, however, confrontation may arise, in some cases leading the caregiver to discharge their dependant back to seven days a week home care. On the hospital statistics, such a discharge may seem a success, but in reality it is more a mixture of victory and failure.

Caregiving and the Breakdown of Care

Finally, I should like to turn to the breakdown of caring. What events lead to the decision that care is transferred from families to institutions, and at what point does informal care give way to formal care? Perhaps the first point to bear in mind is the relative discrepancy between those elderly mentally infirm living alone and those living with others.

Numerous studies have attested to the differential vulnerability of the elderly living alone to being placed in institutional care: those living alone are more likely to be admitted to institutional care, and less likely to be discharged back to the community (Ross and Kedward, 1977; Turner and Sternberg, 1978; Bergmann *et al.*, 1978). Some studies, however, have found social isolation of less relevance to hospital admission than admission to residential care (Gillis *et al.*, 1982). Gaspar (1980) has suggested that the protective influence of living with others may be less for elderly dementing men than it is for women. Giving-up is likely to be related to the elderly dementing person living on their own, so that continuous supervision is not possible without major changes in life-style for the primary supporters, and possibly also to being male, perhaps because their behavioural disturbance is harder for wives or daughters to manage. Gilhooley (1984b) has investigated supporters' willingness to continue caring for an elderly dementing relative, and her findings strongly suggest that spouses are much less likely to consider institutional care than children, and that younger-generation supporters, employed and not living with their dementing relative, are more likely to consider institutional care. She also found, like Hirschfeld in a similar study (Hirschfeld, 1981), that a poor relationship in the past significantly reduced the supporters' willingness to continue caring.

To what extent does the supporters' attitude towards institutionalisation actually determine insitutional admission? In one of our own studies, mentioned in the previous chapter, we interviewed 128 supporters of elderly mentally infirm people referred to daycare services. At the initial interview, we asked whether the supporter felt able to continue caring as they were, and also whether, if there were further deterioration, they would consider long-term care in a home or hospital. Some 70 per cent of those patients whose supporters felt unable to continue coping were in long-term care six months later, and only 20 per cent remained in the community. In addition, 67 per cent of the dependants of those supporters who were unsure were also in long-term care by six months, and 20 per cent remained at home. Of those supporters who felt able to continue caring, 60 per cent were still doing so six months later. With regard to considering long-term care, 70 per cent said they would do so, if there were further deterioration, 20 per cent would not, and 10 per cent did not know. Although only 11 per cent of those who originally would not consider long-term care had 'given up' six months later, almost half (49 per cent) of those saying they would consider long-term care had indeed given up. Evidently attitudes and expectations about continuing the caring role are predictive of future behaviour as a carer.

We also found that, as a group, spouses were much less likely to consider long-term care, and were more likely to feel able to continue in their caring role than other relatives. Only one out of 48 spouses (2 per cent) felt unable to continue caring, though 27 (55 per cent) would consider long-term care in the future, usually if they felt unable to cope with the problems; this contrasts with 57 of the 72 other relatives (79 per cent) who were willing to consider long-term care, and 10 out of 72 (14 per cent) who felt unable to continue caring. In the younger group of supporters, we found that expectations of giving up were more directed to changes in the dependant, for example, if they became more deteriorated, if they became more difficult, etc., while for most spouses, these expectations were usually related to failings within the supporter, e.g. 'not being up to it' any more, failing health, not able to give the necessary help, etc.

Unlike Gilhooley (1984b), we found some relationship between measures of strain and emotional upset and willingness to give up caring, but we found little evidence that strain or emotional distress actually predicted outcome of day-hospital care. Table 6.1 indicates the scores of supporters on the strain scale, the general health questionnaire (GHQ) (a measure of emotional symptomatology, Goldberg, 1978), the problem checklist score and an index of formal support received, according to their dependant's outcome. Details of the measures can be found in the appendix.

Table 6.1: Relationship Between Supporter Strain and Outcome at Six Months from a Sample of Consecutive Referrals for Psychogeriatric Day Care

| | Average score of supporter, when dependant: | | |
	Still in the community $n = 58$	Institutionalised $n = 37$	Died $n = 11$
Professional support	2.8	3.5	2.7
No. of problems	10.0	25.2	24.7
Strain	12.1	14.8	14.0
Distress (as reported by the caregiver on the GHQ)	10.3	13.6	9.3

By using analysis of covariance, it is possible to examine the association between differing outcomes and differing degrees of strain and distress, independently of the number of problems faced (which is the covariate) and, similarly, to examine the association between outcomes and differing levels of problems independently of the degree of strain reported (which is then treated as the covariate). The results indicate that it is problems, not strain or distress, which most closely influence subsequent outcome. Although the reported degree of distress and strain is greater in the group whose dependant is subsequently institutionalised, the differences in scores are not large enough to reject the assumption that they are due to chance.

Taking these results together, then, there is evidence to suggest that willingness to continue caring is predictive of continuing caring behaviour. Such behaviour is not greatly influenced by the strain and morale of the supporter, which does not seem to be predictive of supporters giving up caring. From Table 6.1, it is also apparent that the receipt of professional/formal support is not a significant mediator preventing insitutionalisation, though the problems presented by the dependant clearly are. As was noted above, it was particularly the case for non-spouse caregivers (the majority of our sample) that expectations of future caring were indeed related to their expectations of future behavioural change/deterioration in their dependant. Unfortunately, our sample of spouses is too small to examine with any certainty whether differences in problem-reporting predicted outcome to the same extent, although in general they appear not to. That is, spouse reports of problems for those subsequently institutionalised were not significantly greater than was the case for those whose partner remained at home with them at the end of the six-month follow-up. For the institutionalised group, average total problem score = 25.1 (s.d. 8.1) n = 11; for those still attending day care and at home group, average total problem score = 20.0 (s.d. 9.1), n = 20; significance of the difference, t = 1.5, not significant. For adult children the respective scores were as follows – parent institutionalised six months later, problem checklist score = 27.6 (s.d. 8.7), n = 24; parents at home, and still attending day care, problem score = 15.3 (s.d. 9.2), n = 12, significance of the difference, t = 3.7, $p < 0.01$.

Summary

The results from both our own and others' research point to the complexity of the relationship between stress and strain in caregiving. The sex of the caregiver, and the quality of the past and present relationship seem to influence the amount of strain experienced by caregivers. The presence, but not necessarily the degree of dementia, is an important factor in determining strain. Means of handling the caregiving situation seem to play an important role in mitigating strain, and strategies that involve distancing or disengaging from interpersonal demands as well as those that reflect the adoption of a more indirect care-managing role seem to be associated with lower levels of reported strain.

Finally, there is no clear evidence that levels of reported strain do in fact influence the commitment to maintaining community care. This finding is of particular importance, since it suggests that intervention to alleviate the strain on supporters may not lead to differences in the family's willingness or ability to continue to care. If it is the sense of commitment to caring, irrespective of the strains imposed by such a commitment, that primarily determines outcome, then research and intervention studies need to elucidate the differential links that contribute to strain and commitment. For example, it may be that male supporters are both under less strain from and less committed to caregiving: furthermore, while children and spouse caregivers may not differ in their level of reported strain, they may differ significantly in the extent of their commitment. As a result, different circumstances may operate to produce a breakdown in care for each of these respective groups. The complex links that sustain or lead to the breakdown of the caring relationship between dementia victims and their supporters will no doubt receive further research attention. At present we have several leads, but it would be premature to consider that these can be drawn together into a coherent picture. In particular, a major question-mark hangs over the role that current formal service provision plays. It is sobering that there is so little research support for its impact on alleviating strain or enhancing the commitment to care.

7 COMMUNITY CARE: A REVIEW OF SOME OF THE ISSUES

The existence of long waiting lists for institutional care, the prevalence of high levels of distress amongst caring families, and the financial constraints currently prevailing on community services all demonstrate the difficulties society faces in managing its elderly mentally infirm citizens.

One carer wrote recently: 'it is no exaggeration to say that I would not leave an animal alone to suffer the loneliness, the pain, the anxiety that those two old ladies bore', speaking of her own mother and mother-in-law (Jeanette Bramley, *Guardian,* Monday, 15 August 1983). Another case also reported in the *Guardian* on 13 September 1983, begins: 'A devoted husband killed his 72-year-old senile wife when her nagging became unbearable . . . he cared for her and nursed her under a considerable burden, until 13th October last year when he finally snapped and killed her.' Other cases of extreme strain have been reported in an article in the *Sunday Times,* 2 January 1983; for example, a woman who pushed her mother downstairs after ploys such as leaving the light off had failed to bring about her death by accident.

These 'granny battering' horror stories make a point, but they are overshadowed by the everyday deprivations and hassles which many, if not the majority of carers face, and which make up the background of community care. Of course, attempts are being made to develop innovatory projects which may assist in the community care of the elderly mentally infirm (cf. Age Concern's *Mental Health in Old Age: a Collection of Projects,* 1983). But voluntary schemes and service innovations may do little more than offer palliative solutions without producing any major assistance in day-to-day caring. For example, of 38 day centres for the elderly mentally infirm set up by voluntary agencies, only four were open for more than three days a week and most only one day a week (Age Concern, 1983).

In one recent Swedish study, family members of patients admitted for psychogeriatric care were asked if they thought anything could have been done to prevent their relatives' admission. Invariably they answered negatively (Adolfsson *et al.,* 1980). The same authors have stated elsewhere that 'in Sweden, where large resources are available for welfare and hospital care, it can be expected that most patients with severe dementia are admitted to institutions' (Adolfsson *et al.*, 1981). As was noted in Chapter 3, the Newcastle follow-up studies clearly indicated that institutional care was the most likely outcome for demented persons living in the community.

These authors concluded 'unlike mentally healthy old people and the large majority of those with functional syndromes, who can continue to live at home even when of very advanced age, the majority of the mentally deteriorated aged eventually need constant supervision, which can usually only be given in some kind of institutional setting' (Kay *et al.*, 1970).

Such positions challenge the feasibility of alternative viable caring systems, and place the central issue of community care as the extent to which there exists any real intermediary between the transition from family care to institutional care. Neither the statutory services nor families seem to be able to sustain in the community those elderly mentally infirm people who maintain a separate household. Those who currently exist in this situation remain vulnerable and, it would seem, incapable of being supported with any degree of physical and personal comfort, for any extended period of time.

Dementia, Self-maintenance and Personal Responsibility

As has been pointed out in earlier chapters, the dementing person is rarely cognisant of the extent of his or her own failings, and the decline of insight seems generally directly proportionate to the decline in self-maintenance skills. Indeed, there is often reluctance and refusal to accept external offers of assistance. The need for help and the accompanying incompetence is on such a grand scale that most of the efforts of caregivers to help with daily living tasks represent direct and unambiguous expressions of the dementing individual's personal incompetence. As a care recipient, the dementing person is most often unable and unwilling to share the perspective of caregivers. This lack of reciprocity is itself unrewarding and occasionally aversive to the caregiver, whose thankless caregiving behaviour may only be sustained by the internal rewards of doing one's duty, remaining faithful to one's partner, or fulfilling professional expectations. At the same time, social isolation as a result of caregiving may attenuate the possibility of receiving rewards and reinforcement for other behaviours incompatible with caregiving, 'enmeshing' the carer into a pattern of unrelieved caregiving. Such impersonal reinforcement for caregiving is ecologically unusual, since most naturally arising caring relationships seem presaged upon the experience of external interpersonal reinforcement. The strains imposed by this type of caring relationship are understandably great, perhaps particularly for those who do receive reinforcement from alternative behaviours, and for whom the conflicts of caring are greatest (cf. Johnson, 1983).

The extent to which the dementing person is unable to relate to his or her immediate physical and personal environment means that the engagement with family and neighbourhood is tenuous, at best. The sense of belonging is slowly disrupted; witness the poignant requests to go home now, to join mother who is waiting for them and the misrecognition of family and friends. This inability to retain consciously information by which one may locate the social and physical self serves to disrupt links with the interpersonal environment, so that it becomes increasingly meaningless to view such individuals as an active element of any social network.

Finally, the growing failure to form, or retain, plans of action and goals reflects a fundamental decline in personal responsibility and intentionality, such that the dementing individual cannot be held truly accountable for his or her reactions and behaviour. This failure of mental competence may or may not be legally ratified, but it renders dubious the view that the individual personally 'owns' their own household. Yet very often there remains extreme concern for personal belongings. Others may be accused of stealing money, hiding clothing, or locking away valuables. The anxiety to retain one's bearings, to hang on to those external cues which help prompt a sense of identity may be apparent even in quite severely demented individuals. This leads to a natural reluctance to dispossess the elderly mentally frail of such powerful sources of security in exchange for the more physically, but less psychologically secure environment of an institution. The contrast between the evident value of home for the dementing person and their incompetence to maintain a house provides yet one more dilemma, uniquely characterising the position of the carer and their elderly dementing relative living in the community.

Caring and Responsibility   *dependence ?*
                                 independence •

Taking care of, and taking responsibility for, the elderly dementing person is an important issue which deserves careful consideration. In the previous section, the problems of caring for dementing people were outlined in terms of the lack of a shared perspective of need, the lack of external rewards for the caring relationship, the lack of personal relatedness to the social environment of family and neighbourhood, and the lack of personal responsibility and accountability. The consequence of these problems is that carers must themselves determine the extent of their caregiving responsibilities.   *y of care?*

The entry into a caregiving relationship with a dementing relative usually involves a transitional period for family members, and thus the distinction between past relationships and current caregiving may be one which is imprecisely realised by both partners. The behavioural and attitudinal changes that occur during this transition may be very much the result of a one-sided recognition of the need to change by the caregiver. Before any signs of overt mental incompetence, there may have been a mutually satisfactory increase in helpfulness by the carer towards the parent or spouse, because of physical limitations associated with restricted mobility and other physical ills. Such an intermediary stage may be interspersed between independence of both carer and caregiver and the dependency brought on by mental incompetence, which can soften the transition in roles. Mutual helping, particularly in the case of husband and wife, may mean that interdependency slowly shifts to dependency. On the other hand, mental deterioration may be the primary reason for a disjunctive move from an independent relationship to that of one-sided dependency, particularly in the case of adult children caring for and supervising a physically fit, 60 or 70-year-old dementing parent.

The increase of supervisory caregiving behaviour entails not only the provision of service behaviours to supplement the disabilities of the dependant (help with shopping, cooking, dressing and bathing), but also the provision of restraining or correcting behaviours to reduce the occurrence of non-adaptive behaviours, such as wandering, inappropriate undressing, verbal abuse, misrecognitions and misperceptions. Such supervisory caregiving behaviour entails an attitude of feeling responsible for the dementing person, and it seems likely that the extent of such supervisory caregiving is directly proportional to the supporter's felt sense of responsibility for their dependant.

The issue that this poses is the extent to which such responsibility entails the sense of ownership of the bed. When the dementing person lives with their primary supporter (i.e. the individual engaging most frequently in both service behaviours and restraining or correcting behaviours – supervisory caregiving), then the acceptance of responsibility, both personally and socially, seems to involve implicit ownership of the dementing person's bed. When the primary supporter does not live with the dementing person, their supervisory caregiving will be more often than not on a lesser scale, and there may be then considerable uncertainty as to who owns the bed.

The concepts of taking responsibility for the person, and maintaining a bed, contrast in an exaggerated form the personal and impersonal elements of caring. Yet the extension of the concept of 'the bed' beyond the area of health and welfare administration to encompass the area of interpersonal community can be useful for a number of reasons. First, it recognises that where the dementing person sleeps (i.e. is not actively cared for) is of fundamental importance to the division between community and institutional services. Second, it makes explicit the increasingly external nature of caring – the person within being less and less evident, and their physical presence being more obvious and significant than their psychological presence. Many supporters, as research described in earlier chapters suggests, actively disengage from personal caring, using strategies variously described as 'distancing' or 'ignoring', and many comment that their mother/father/wife/husband has 'died', and for this they mourn, while continuing to care for the impersonal needs of their dependant. Third, it seems to reflect accurately the real links that exist between the provision of institutional care and community care for the elderly mentally infirm – that is, the explicit need for 'continual' supervision. As was pointed out in Chapter 5, the majority of carers looking after their elderly mentally infirm relative felt they could not be left alone for even one hour. Such perceived need for care is implicitly behind the provision of long-term institutional beds for dementing patients, yet clearly is applicable to the situation of many carers in the community.

Beds and Responsibility

If one accepts an equivalence between taking responsibility for the care of a dementing person and maintaining their bed, then it becomes possible to view issues of responsibility as those involved in accepting ownership of the person's bed. This acceptance of ownership is clearly easier for those family carers who share the same household than it is for those who visit and support; the reciprocal condition applies to the state welfare services in accepting ownership of beds. Those elderly mentally infirm people maintaining or failing to maintain an independent household are more likely to be taken as the state's responsibility, whereas those sharing their household, and thus having a responsible person in the household to maintain the bed, will be less readily taken on as the state's responsibility.

There has been for many years a progressive rise in the number of elderly living alone: in 1951, 13 per cent of the over-65s lived alone, in 1961, 22 per cent, and in 1981, the figure was 35 per cent. While the majority have children and are visited by the family, their physical separateness is of crucial significance when the person begins dementing. The absence of a 'prompter' to cue daily behaviours may result in an earlier and clearer recognition of incompetence and non-responsibility, the existence of need and an unallocated responsibility to sustain or maintain a bed. This need to determine ownership of the bed is illustrated by recent experience in the Japanese welfare system. Although the 'vulnerable' group of elderly people living on their own is much smaller in Japan than in Britain, there too the numbers are growing. According to national figures, in 1969, 5 per cent of the over-65s lived alone, while by 1979, 8.5 per cent did so (Maeda, 1978; Ikegami, 1982). This group is inevitably over-represented in institutional settings, hospitals and homes for the aged, as in Britain. However, because of a widespread tradition in Far East Asia that elderly parents are maintained by the children, the issue of need for institutional care for parents whose bed is maintained within a joint household poses serious problems. An increasingly common response has been the 'division of household', a unique administrative procedure which 'produces for form's sake a new household with only a single old person who has been living with his adult child in a joint household' (Makizano, 1978). Such procedures illustrate the capacity of state welfare services to temporarily own 'community' beds, at an administrative level. It can also be argued that such ownership can also be extended without such explicit formality by the concentration of statutory welfare services on maintaining an elderly infirm person at home.

Thus, by providing services explicitly to maintain a community bed, an implicit ownership and transfer of care responsibility can arise that demands an eventual transfer of the bed into an institution, when the statutory welfare services can no longer manage to maintain the community location of the bed. In this context, it is interesting to review one of the few randomised controlled trials of community care, carried out in the United States, and reported by Blenkner and her colleagues. In this study, an experimental group of 76 elderly people were assigned to one of four highly trained caseworkers for protective services, while 88 clients were handled through usual casework agencies. The experimental group received more services, and more than one-third were institutionalised within one year; in contrast, the controls received less services and only one-fifth were institutionalised (Blenkner *et al.*, 1971). A significant proportion, though by no means all of these elderly people, were mentally impaired. The extent to which statutory welfare services may 'take over' the bed can be seen as contributing directly to the transfer of that bed to an institutional setting.

The counterpart of this statutory system, for families, is when the family supporter invests an increasing amount of time providing services to maintain the relative in his or her bed, until this system cannot be managed, and transfer of the bed to the supporter's home is accomplished. However, it is doubtful if family carers and statutory services have an equivalence of resources, and although institutional care may be rationed, once accomplished, it will rarely produce for the institutional caregivers the strains which fall upon those family members who transfer their dependant's bed into their own household. Thus in our own study of 129 supporters of the elderly mentally infirm, 83.3 per cent of those who made such household alterations had their dependant in institutional care some six months later – in contrast to 34 per cent of those who made no such alterations.

The potential for statutory services working in the community to take on responsibility for maintaining community beds, their difficulties in doing so, and the likely costs that may arise from eventual transfer to institutions has led to a reaction against such direct service giving. The British government response, evident in the

White Paper entitled *Growing Older* and in the commissioned Barclay Report, has been to advocate an 'enabling' as distinct from a 'delivery' role for these services, and speaks of developing a 'partnership' with informal care networks in the community (DHSS, 1981; Barclay, 1982).

This reluctance to risk owning and maintaining community beds is justified by the dubious notion of facilitating community care networks, a concept which is increasingly being criticised as unrealistic and unworkable in present-day society.

Community Care Networks and Caregiving Behaviour

Some of the most trenchant criticisms of this concept of community care networks have recently been made by Allan (1983) in his discussion of the Barclay Report (1982). He argues that 'community' is increasingly defined, not by any geographical features, but in terms of social networks. However, Allan points out that 'the social conditions that led to the development of extensive local networks have disappeared . . . no longer are people trapped by their locality in quite the way they were' and, as a result, there is in reality 'little evidence to support the idea that non-kin play a significant part in informal caring' (Allan, 1983).

Pointing out that friends, neighbours and non-primary kin (that is, excluding parents, siblings and children) form relationships which rarely involve the concept of domestic intervention and, even less often, personal 'hands-on' assistance, Allan argues that most caregiving arises from the activities of one or more close relatives, usually female. Moreover, he argues, the idea that these other relationships can be enabled to perform necessary caregiving behaviour implies 'that all forms of relationships can readily be converted into caring ones'. But, as he points out, 'in normal routine life they are not created for this sort of work'.

This erroneous model of community networks fails to address the very real issues that exist in community care, namely, that the great bulk of informal caring is done by female close relatives, and that it is these primary supporters who in reality are not a 'caring network', but individuals struggling with providing supervisory and supportive care to relatives with whom they have shared a significant proportion of their life.

As was pointed out in Chapter 4, many of the services provided by the statutory sector do not supply more than a fraction of the caregiving behaviours required to maintain an elderly demented person in the community, and, as is apparent from the above, informal networks are unlikely to do any better. The perception of what is needed is, as Gilbert Smith has pointed out in his book, *Social Need* (Smith, 1980, pp. 65–85), largely determined by the practices in which the need-supplying agent or agency engages. There is precious little similarity between the practices of the primary supporter of an elderly dementing person and the practices of the statutory services, outside of institutions. This gap between practices is mirrored in a gap between the respective perceptions of need. Caregivers themselves seem to recognise this, since they very rarely can offer advice to the statutory services as to what help or advice could be offered. In our sample of 129 supporters of elderly mentally infirm referrals for day care, described in Chapter 5, the reponse to our question 'what sort of help or advice do you think will be helpful?' was restricted to such comments as 'help me to be more patient', 'they might suggest something I could be doing', or more typically, 'I don't know, I don't think there would be anything'.

Caring for the Carers

One increasing response to these problems may be summarised as directing care to the primary caregivers, principally in the form of relieving the burden of constant caregiving through sitting services, day centres/hospitals and through self-help support groups (Age Concern, 1983). These responses originate as much from the voluntary sector as they do from the statutory services. Attempts to evaluate the impact of such relief-giving services are limited in both number and scope. Psychogeriatric day hospitals seem to lose more than half of their dementing attenders after six months (Gilleard, 1984b), largely to institutional care. As was noted in Chapter 6, while strain and willingness to continue caring are related, it is the latter which primarily determines the breakdown of family care. Thus, even if these respite services do relieve strain, they may do little to reduce the probability that caring at home will break down. Bergmann *et al.* (1978) have clearly demonstrated that those living alone, even with day care and community health and social services, are still highly likely to be institutionalised. Of course, it should be pointed out that other studies have not been quite so definite regarding the significance of 'living alone'. Thus Greene and Timbury (1979) failed to observe any relationship between living arrangements and outcome of day hospital attendance for dementing patients. Gilleard and Watt (1982) found some evidence of differential outcomes according to living arrangements – notably, that 81 per cent of those dementing patients living with spouses, in contrast to 54 per cent of those living alone or with children, were still attending day hospital six months after starting attendance.

While caring and respite services for the carers may be inherently desirable, it is still not clear whether such services have any impact on the maintenance of community beds for the elderly mentally infirm.

Caregiving, Need and Responsibility

One feature of respite services is that they are designed to reduce the amount of caregiving behaviour – both supportive and supervisory – that carers engaged in. As Chapter 5 showed, the need to give constant supervision is the single most important problem for carers, and thus there appears to be some appropriate matching of needs through such provision. However, one may ask what effect altering the amount of caregiving has, not on strain, but on commitment to care.

Festinger and Carlsmith performed an experiment which has become something of a classic in social psychology. It has been summarised as follows:

> College students were brought one at a time to a small room to work for half an hour on two very dull and repetitive tasks [stacking spools and turning pegs]. After completing the tasks, some of the students were offered one dollar to go into the waiting room and tell the next subject that the tasks were fun and interesting. Other students were offered twenty dollars to do the same thing . . . Later all of the students were asked for their actual opinions of the tasks . . . The students who had been paid only one dollar stated that they had, in fact, enjoyed the task. But students who had been paid twenty dollars did not (Hilgard, Atkinson and Atkinson, 1975, p. 539).

The explanation was developed in terms of cognitive dissonance theory, which, in its simplified form, states that people maintain attitudes which reduce inconsistencies between their actions and their thoughts.

By giving care, then, one might expect that the belief that such caregiving is one's responsibility would be maintained, and even enhanced. Given the opportunity not to give care, or reducing caregiving behaviour, may thus reduce the feeling of responsibility, and alter perceptions of need. Similarly, not being able to meet what one perceives to be needed may also alter the feeling or attitude of responsibility, whereas being able to give care success-fully and as one perceives it to be needed may enhance this attitude of responsibility. Thus these three elements of the caring relation-ship stand in reciprocal relationship to one another. Figure 7.1 provides a simplified diagrammatic model of this situation.

Figure 7.1: The Elements of Care

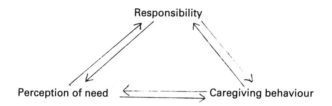

The family caregiver who lives with the dementing person is likely to perceive a wider range of needs, engage in more supervisory and supportive caregiving and feel a greater responsibility for the main-tenance of their dependant and their bed. Intervention in this system may, by reducing caregiving behaviour, alter the attitude of responsibility – producing the risk of services being seen to 'take over' care. It is equally possible, however, that intervention can enhance caregiving behaviour – leading to a better match between need and met need, and ultimately enhancing responsibility. The recent study by Greene *et al.* (1983) demonstrating that teaching reality-orientation skills to supporters increased their sense of coping illustrates this type of effect.

One crucial element, therefore, in this sytem is the actual range of caregiving behaviours available to the carer. Limitations in caregiving may arise from physical ill-health (particularly with elderly spouses or siblings), lack of time (particularly with married daughters) or lack of skills (particularly with male supporters). Such imbalance may lead to alterations in the sense of responsibility or alterations in perception of need. The latter is illustrated in Gilhooley's (1981) 'ignoring' strategy and Johnson and Catelona's (1982) 'distancing' technique. The former will of course be seen when supporters actively seek to transfer responsibility outside the household. In the absence of care networks, this means transferring responsibility to the statutory services.

Such a model has limitations, and ignores the temporal dimension of change that is so important in dementia. Balanced systems may develop, only to be threatened by the dependant's deterioration – enhancing need beyond the range of current caregiving practice, or enhancing current caregiving practice beyond its self-perceived effectiveness – or by changes in the supporters' circumstances – e.g. health, other family relationships changing, especially the marital relationship which may also affect caregiving practice and effectiveness. Such changes may then be met by alterations in responsibility, developing more caregiving skills or denying problems and thus altering perceptions of need.

Those whose time is their own, spouses and retired siblings living with their dependant, may feel that there is unlimited scope for increasing caregiving behaviours and thus may respond by increasingly forming what Johnson and Catelona described as 'enmeshed' relationships with their dependant. The man who took his wife out of day care illustrates this situation. Married and/or working daughters may not be in this position, and thus provide a more vulnerable care system.

Finally, 'need' within this system may be quite different from 'need' as described in social-policy terms, since need to maintain or sustain the person at home will involve the carer's perception of what the 'person at home' is. Thus the need may be to keep mother behaving as 'mother', and to reduce or minimise evidence of the changes that threaten this social/interpersonal self: similarly, with husbands, wives and sisters. The quality of the past relationship may then impose constraints on what the supporter needs to do to maintain the person – quite distinct from simply maintaining the bed. Such a view of the other and the need to sustain this interpersonally important self will not – cannot – be shared by the agents of either voluntary or statutory services. This may enhance the difficulty of transferring responsibility for meeting the dependant's needs, as seen by their relative, onto an impersonal service agent. The quality of the past relationship will also produce in those who engage in caregiving variable responses to their responsibility. They may not have liked or got on with the dependant, and thus not feel that their dependant's personal needs require the level of attention that those who have been closer feel. As Hirschfeld (1981) found, however, this may not lead to any significant loss in the degree of assumed responsibility, but rather a more restricted or impersonal style of caregiving.

Summary

The issues discussed in this chapter seem to the author to require, first, a realistic recognition of what community care means in practice. It involves a limited, often individual task, with external service influences only marginally touching upon the nature of the caregiver's role. It can be seen as made up of three principal elements: (a) responsibility lacking in the dependant and required of the carer; (b) need perceived by the carer, yet not expressed by the dependant; and (c) caregiving behaviour both supervisory, preventing disturbed and dangerous behaviour, and supportive, providing assistance for impaired or non-existent self-help skills, all of which converge upon each other in reciprocal relationships to form a focused and self-regulating circle of care. As the dementia progresses, both behavioural and cognitive readjustments are called for, involving changes in perceived need, responsibility and caregiving as the emphasis becomes increasingly one of maintaining a bed, rather than maintaining a person. Such a shift requires a reliance upon internal reinforcement, as external reciprocity declines, and caring for begins to pre-empt caring about. This situation is less easily responded to by existing community services, which, if they do take over, are likely sooner or later to transfer the locus of bed maintenance from the community to an institutional setting, where caregiving more closely approximates that offered by the living-in supporter.

Intervention may as easily disrupt this circle of care as strengthen and sustain it, and it is only by the careful appraisal of the three elements – caregiving, perceived need and responsibility – that appropriate decisions regarding professional involvement can be made. Interventions which fail to consult properly with the primary caregiver are clearly more likely to be unsuccessful. In the final chapter, discussion will be focused upon an appropriate set of goals for an integrated psychogeriatric (dementia) service.

8 LOOKING TO THE FUTURE: A PROPOSED MODEL OF CARE

To some extent we are all 'living with dementia'. Socio-economic and technological changes which have developed over the last two hundred years have resulted in a demographic structure which now ensures that it is no longer rare to reach one's eightieth birthday. This inevitably exposes more people to the deteriorative processes that constitute brain ageing. Not only does the brain, like any other bodily organ, become vulnerable to failures in self-maintenance, but it does so from an inherently more vulnerable status than most other bodily organs. To use a popular computer analogy, it cannot renew its hardware: once lost or dysfunctional, nerve cells are not replaced. The extent of this neuronal fallout over the lifespan remains an issue for debate (Hanley, 1974; Ball, 1977; Brodie, 1978), but its existence is undeniable. While there may be considerable neuronal redundancy – in the sense that normal brain function may not be greatly compromised by some degree of cell loss – the extent to which neuronal cells require continual complex metabolic activity to maintain their unique properties of excitability and conductivity means that they are at risk of developing errors across numerous fronts. Indeed, for 80 or 90 years they must replace different types of proteins, maintain intracellular transport systems, synthesise complex amino acids and of course retain their structural integrity.

Even when such long-serving systems remain error-free, other non-neuronal support systems must also retain their integrity of function – the vascular system in particular may prove a potential source of failure, leading to strokes, small or large, causing neuronal damage; the glial cells and the cellular structure of the cerebral meninges may develop abnormal proliferative dysfunction, leading to tumour growth, and so on. For such reasons it may be of little value to separate abnormal ageing of brain functions from some assumed normal ageing process. Ageing is not a benign process and it seems equally unrealistic to dub age-associated memory and intellectual losses as benign. Of course, variations in the rate and extent of these maintenance failures in differing neuronal subsystems may produce differential trajectories of failure in cognitive performance, and there is an enormous need to develop greater empirical understanding of the mechanisms by which different maintenance failures arise. The essential point is, however, that by separating out a group of ageing individuals whose brains are deemed abnormally aged, or dementing, we may be creating artificial dichotomies which in reality cut off such individuals from the common and universal plight of our own ageing, and which perhaps serve to defend our own vulnerable selves from facing up to a common biological fate. To say this is not to say that everyone, if they were to live long enough, would become demented in the *same way* as those who dement in their fifties, sixties, seventies or eighties. Breakaway ageing of certain neural systems may be more common in dementias of early onset (e.g. the cholinergic system in Alzheimer's dementia), while similar 'breakaway' ageing of other systems may be less intellectually devastating (e.g. the dopaminergic system in Parkinson's disease), and most people may suffer less by a more even distribution of ageing changes within the brain. Nevertheless, there is consistent evidence that, with increasing age, mental incompetence characterises an ever-growing minority. One recent New Zealand community study observed that of those in their nineties more than 40 per cent demonstrated mental incompetence of a degree found in only some 2 per cent of people in their sixties (Campbell *et al.*, 1983).

If, then, we recognise the common problem of maintaining a continuity of self in the face of our biological ageing, it becomes possible to consider how elderly people are best served when faced with a crumbling neurological substructure and a declining ability to master the resources of their physical and social environment. Perhaps the best answer is to protect such individuals as far as possible from failure, and when failure occurs, to help cushion the impact of that failure. As the integrity of the self declines further, such response to these personal needs may become less necessary, and it may then be of more value to expend psychological effort in comforting those for whom loss of the person is hardest to bear. Meantime, as only the less personal characteristics of the individual remain, the caregiving task becomes increasingly one of providing physical ease and reducing physical disease.

Such a model is obviously beset with problems of definition, and the next section of this chapter is concerned with identifying these definitional problems and the dilemmas they produce. Although I do not believe that any absolute solutions can be found, I would like to hope that ideological and empirical approaches can be merged to help elucidate some of the options that may be worth pursuing.

Identification of Dementia

The 'demand'-based model of health and social-service care may not serve the elderly population very well and many have argued for an active case-finding and screening approach to service provision for the elderly (e.g. Williamson, 1981). In contrast to screening for prodromal signs of 'pre-dementia', it is perhaps most important that as many as possible of the people demonstrating clinically recognisable dementia are recognised (diagnosed) at as early a stage as possible.

Thus the 'need' may not be for any increasing sophistication in the use of psychological, biochemical or neurophysiological indices to pick up 'pre-dementing' states, but an increase in the effective recognition of existing established dementing processes, marked by memory failure, difficulties in maintaining a household, and some degree of impaired 'reality' orientation. Such clinical signs can be based upon any of the present 'mental status' questionnaires (cf. Gurland, 1980) combined with information from family members or neighbours regarding the at-risk person's ability to manage everyday tasks (cf. Kellett *et al.*, 1975).

Such case-finding could be made the responsibility of a community nurse or health visitor specialising in work with the elderly in a group practice or health centre, and initially focusing upon the over-75s. Those identified as probably dementing (cf. Gurland, 1980) could then be visited by the doctor, and where the change was recent (i.e. within the last three months), further investigations, including geriatric and psychogeriatric specialist referral, could be initiated. Once the impairment is confirmed by the doctor and its presence established for at least six months, the need for community-based health and social services investigations could then be considered.

The extent to which reversible non-neuropathological factors contribute to the appearance of dementia was touched upon in Chapter 2. The results of such investigations strongly suggest that in the over-70s those individuals with a clinical diagnosis of dementia will rarely have a reversible pathology accounting for their mental deterioration, especially if it has been evident for an extended period of time. The emphasis on such pathologies – accounting for less than 10 per cent of elderly people with dementia – can easily lead to the rejection of the vast bulk of persistently and progressively impaired individuals whose needs extend well beyond laboratory investigations and computerised tomographic scanning. It is only when dementia leads to neglect and lack of continued medical and psychiatric involvement that the so-called dangers of labelling arise. If the identification and diagnosis of dementia leads to positive action and sustained concern, such changes can largely be avoided. Identification should thus be a positive step in instituting a course of management based upon the accurate ascertainment of mental incompetence and decline of personal responsibility.

Action after Identification

Elderly people living on their own with a clinically established dementia are not in a position to maintain for any length of time an independent household. Consultation between community services and those family members actively caring for such individuals should focus on long-term management plans which must involve a reasoned judgement and allocation of responsibility – deciding if family carers wish to accept responsibility and, if need be, bring their relative into their own household, or whether they wish to be supportive caregivers but with the statutory services taking principal responsibility for the elderly dementing person. Such discussions following identification require an agreed 'care-manager' who will take or share the principal responsibility for future developments. The difficulties for the statutory services is that unless such an individual has access to residential beds, his or her ability to manage the care system effectively may be very limited. At present, for example, general practitioners and field social workers are not in such a position.

Elderly dementing people living in shared households are not in the position of having to maintain an independent household. The identification of such individuals obviously involves intrusion into the carer's household by the statutory services, and discussion of long-term management may not be so easily broached. The explicit responsibility for the dementing person may not necessarily be a subject for debate at this stage, but the opportunity to discuss the situation can be taken, the needs of the supporter identified, and a basis for sustained contact between family and services negotiated. The aim is obviously to enable the supporters to manage effectively their caring activities.

Care-managing

The work of Archbold (1981), referred to in Chapter 5, illustrates the separate behaviours involved in 'caregiving' and 'care-managing'. The former, hands-on service, is seen as inherently more stressful and probably more a 'female' behavioural style, one which involves the provision of supportive caregiving (washing, dressing, rising and transferring, toiletting, feeding, etc. – which are commonly seen as 'nursing' activities). In the case of caregiving to dementing elderly relatives, it also involves a supervisory monitoring of potentially hazardous 'error-prone' behaviours, and may thus require the caregiver to interfere with the dementing person's behaviour, with the potential for generating considerably more strain than that originating from carrying out purely supportive caregiving, as was shown in the studies described in Chapter 5.

The difficulties in providing substitutive caregiving relationships, commented upon critically by Allan (1983), are the difficulties of providing substitutive caregiving behaviours. Opportunities for care-managing depend upon identifying the best means of delivering such substitutive acts to minimise individual supporter exhaustion. At one level, supportive caregiving is more easily substituted than supervisory caregiving. District nurses may help dress, toilet, bathe and wash the dependant. However, a major problem that arises is the enforced recognition of incompetence that this potentially entails for the dementing person. In some cases, a non-family member is less threatening – there is less need to preserve a continuous competent self, and previous experience of being nursed may facilitate the constant body intimacy involved, when the caregiver is demonstrably 'a professional nurse'.

Other substitutive services – cleaning, laundry, shopping, sitting – can be seen as lying within the province of the home-help service. Unfortunately, the provision of such services is rarely made when the elderly person lives with adult children. More problematic is the supervisory monitoring which may occupy considerably more of the carer's time than that spent in supportive caregiving. The use of day care as a means of relieving carers from full-time supervisory care and the development of sitting services, in evenings and at week-ends, may all be seen as means of providing substitutive supervisory care. The latter, in particular, has developed from voluntary rather than statutory schemes, and is consequently an uneven provision in the country as a whole.

However, one drawback to the institution of substitutive services is the extent to which they erode the commitment to care or 'sense of responsibility' and disturb the balance between need, care and responsibility within the family care system that may have evolved prior to case-identification, simply by reducing the extent of the carer's caregiving involvement – and implicitly, and most impor-tantly, reducing their care-managing role. The early institution of substitutive service resources, which can be jointly managed by the family and professional carers, may avoid some of the problems that can currently be observed within more crisis-directed service systems – namely, families giving up shortly after day care or other services are started, or day patients dropping out because of in-adequate preparation, or appropriateness of the placement, etc.

The development of 'packages' of substitutive service provisions is still largely reactive and needs to be made more prescriptive. How that may be achieved depends in great measure upon the develop-ment of an appropriate model of needs that is made available to practitioners.

Needs

A model of 'needs' must centre upon the overall situation of the dementing person. Needs require elucidation, not primarily as ex-pressed personal distress or dissatisfaction, but more as they are mirrored in the responses made towards the dementing person by their carer. This requires an advocate for the patient who is likely to have a continuous knowledge of the person who is dementing, their customary habits and means of adjusting to problems. At the same time, if carers are now having to take on responsibility for the dementing person's behaviour, then their perceptions of need must be acknowledged as primary. There can be little validity to statements such as 'what dementing people need is/are . . .' Their past individuality as seen by the carer needs careful delineation.

The professional should not work only from a purely reactive position – 'what do you want me to do?' Certain goals, however much they may reflect abstract general principles, need to be borne in mind, which entail (a) a recognition of the need for security by maintaining contact with the social and physical environment most likely to have been a continuous element of the dementing person's life-style, (b) recognition of the need to minimise failure of self-maintenance or confrontation with such failures, and (c) provision of adequate bodily comfort.

Finally, the carer's need to manage caring activities must be ascertained. This is of course not a static position, and underlines the necessity for continued contact between the statutory services and the family. The experience of not managing, of failing to cope with the demands of caregiving, may require behavioural intervention (for example, improving caregiving skills), cognitive intervention (altering the perceptions of need), or physical intervention (reducing the level of responsibility for meeting the needs of the dependent relative).

Family Counselling

Since dementia presents a problem of one family member whose behaviour becomes increasingly deficient and defectively controlled, the position of that person within the family becomes an increasingly difficult element within the social life of the family as a whole – a situation arising more quickly and more urgently when the person lives within the same household. The concern for these failings is therefore very often a family concern, that one member is failing to act as they have customarily acted, and thus that their role within the family is increasingly incompetently performed – they are no longer the person they once were.

Thus it is most often other family members, not the dementing person, whose concern is expressed by seeking assistance – most often directed towards the general practitioner. Aside from the problems of examining someone who has not personally sought intervention for themselves, the doctor is also in the position of acting in such a way as to relieve the distress of others over their relative's behaviour.

The patient as a 'third-person' problem is obviously perceived by the family as not fully responsible, and therefore needing their help as agents in receiving medical care. At the same time, it is unlikely that deterioration will have progressed to such a point where the elderly person has given up any attempts at exercising independence and thus presents both as third person and second person to the doctor (what's the matter with you?, what's the matter with her?). This split over 'agency', the part division of responsibility, will have already occurred, and the doctor has to balance these two differing objectives of his consultation.

Under these circumstances, the separate activities of identification and management become especially important. Identification is patient-oriented and family provide only collateral information to reach a formulation. However, if identification leads to a formulation of dementia (that is, a global progressive intellectual and behavioural deterioration), then management becomes increasingly management of a social problem rather than a purely individual one.

The extent to which the implications of dementia can be explored within the family context and the extent to which negotiations over responsibilities can be effectively made between doctor and family depend upon both clinical and interpersonal skill. Such discussion as takes place obviously is set within a temporal framework; not only is there the question of what needs to be done now, but the recognition that circumstances will continue, most probably, to change in the future. Thus, negotiations will need to be part of a continuing partnership between the family and the statutory services.

At this stage, specialists (geriatricians, psychogeriatricians) are most often brought in, not principally as people with special expertise in identification, or as individuals with skills in giving advice, but primarily as owners of resources – most notably psychiatric or geriatric beds or part-beds (that is, day hospital places).

How much further other resource-owning individuals will be called in will depend upon individual circumstances – home helps, incontinence services, district nurses, etc. What is certain is that a form of impersonal prescription is likely to be dispensed to families, much in the way that medications are prescribed as impersonal means of combating an impersonal disease process.

Backing off from the personal dimension is relatively easier in resource-rich areas, and less easy when the services are not available. However, as I tried to intimate in Chapter 4, the sort of services most frequently associated with the elderly infirm are often quite inappropriate for the elderly dementing person, and fail to address the fundamental problem of loss of agency or loss of self that requires recognition and understanding – recognition that others will increasingly have to act as the person responsible for conducting, controlling and supervising the behavioural repertoire of the dementing person, and understanding of the realignments of personal relationships that will inevitably occur as a result.

Working through the complex personal issues of need, responsibility and care-managing with family members is maybe too much to expect of general practitioners, and it could be argued that it requires unique professional counselling skills. Certainly some psychogeriatricians are highly skilled at this task, as well as being owners of invaluable resources which permit them to explore more freely issues of carers giving up or transferring responsibility for maintaining the bed. The principal disadvantages for leaving it to the psychogeriatricians is their relative scarcity, and their almost inevitable link with psychiatric hospital beds or day places. This latter problem deserves some separate consideration.

Psychogeriatrics: Hospital or Residential Services

Psychogeriatricians inherited beds in mental hospitals that were vacated as a result of more active management approaches to inmates with chronic psychiatric disorders. They were also influential in obtaining admission/assessment inpatient units as an active 'upfront' hospital service, and more recently they have increasingly turned to adding on day-hospital units, either purpose-built or converted from existing hospital buildings. All this locates a dementia service within the psychiatric hospital. Geriatricians, on the other hand, serving the physical and social needs of the ill elderly, seem to have had dementia thrust upon them as part of the so-called 'geriatric triad' of ills that, in varying degrees, accompanies their patients into hospital, as harbingers of potential chronicity and long-term bed occupancy.

For many geriatricians, dementia is a frequent, but in some ways 'accompanying' or 'additional' problem, not a central feature of their service – perhaps because the body, not the mind, still largely offers the geriatrician his principal target of care.

It must be asked whether, as the elderly person fails, slowly but surely to cope with independence, choice and self-maintenance, hospital offers any adequate substitution service for that failure; does it cushion that failure in any way? Many of those who advocate community care at least see clearly the inappropriateness of hospital care for the maladies accompanying the deterioration of the self. For in hospital, most of the external cues that might preserve or support the 'historical' self and most aspects of the social environment that might cue appropriate behavioural sequences are simply absent. The skills of doctors and nurses in hospitals are not designed primarily to support a personal system of identity, nor do they validate and sustain fragile elements of a 60- or 70-year life course that has never incorporated communal living in settings for the mentally or physically ill. At best, hospitals may take over the care of an ageing body, the owner of which is accepted as becoming absent and to whom no personal bonds of responsibility can be developed. From this perspective, it would be unrealistic to view such a care system as failing, since the very self to whom personal care had been given is already partially if not totally lost, even to those who could validate that individual's identity. Hospitalisation may then be seen as meeting the personal needs of family carers, and the physical needs of an ageing body.

Yet, particularly for those dementing people who have been living alone, entry to hospital may take place at a point when some personal current relatedness to their home environment remains, in some cases to quite a substantial degree. The alternative to hospital is not an absence of institutional care provision, but a non-hospital environment that offers some kind of home where the person can pass away with the minimum physical distress and maximum psychological security. Homes for the elderly mentally infirm are not popular options (cf. Meacher, 1972), but they could well offer a style of residential care that produces much less of a personal discontinuity than is found in long-stay psychogeriatric wards. To criticise the appropriateness of hospital care should not lead us into imagining that most family care systems are inevitably capable or can be made capable of maintaining dementing people at home until death.

Psychogeriatric services could be provided outwith any psychiatric hospital base by teams working jointly in day centres and homes, with access and ideally control over the running of a general hospital-based psychogeriatric inpatient assessment unit. In an area of 50,000 people, approximately 7,500 will be aged over 65 years. Assuming a 6.5 per cent prevalence figure for dementia (see Chapter 3), around 450 elderly people would be dementing, served by approximately 15 to 20 general practitioners. Approximately one-third (150) will be living alone, and highly likely to move into institutional care during the course of their deterioration (Kay *et al.*, 1970); a further third or less (*c.*120) will be living and being looked after by an elderly spouse; slightly more than one-third (*c.*170) will be living with other relatives. Four 30-bed residential units or homes, and two psychogeriatric day centres, taking up to 50 places per week, could effectively reach the majority of the demented elderly within that population centre, with a 15-bed assessment ward taking in 50 to 60 new 'probable' cases each year, as well as 10 per cent (40–50) of the existing cases in the area, for stays of up to six weeks per year. Given a current provision of 20 residential home places, ten of which will be occupied by mentally infirm persons (Masterton, Holloway and Timbury, 1979; Clarke, Williams and Jones, 1981), five 'psychiatric/psychogeriatric' beds and four or five psychogeriatric day places per 1,000 over 65 years, reflecting current 'norms' (cf. DHSS, 1972; Wattis, Wattis and Arie, 1981), the proposed alternative service would represent 16 residential places per 1,000 people aged 65 or over, 14 day places per 1,000 and 2 psychogeriatric beds per 1,000 over-65s devoted to the elderly mentally infirm. Thus the absolute rise in residential places would be 20 per cent (from current levels of *c.* 15–18 places per 1,000), while day places would have to rise by approximately 300 per cent. Assuming that residential home places represent approximately 60 per cent of the cost of hospital places (cf. Ross, 1976), the likely increase in costs for residential provision would be approximately 13 per cent, while the cost of day centre places would obviously be much greater.

Such a service would nevertheless confer considerable benefits by providing a continuity and comprehensiveness in the care offered to dementing people and their families, and remove the current stigma associated with sending a relative into a mental hospital for the rest of their life. A freer choice for relatives, and a more residential and personalised environment for long-term care, would remove much of the guilt and resulting emotional blackmail that unfortunately characterise current approaches to transferring responsibility from family care to state institutions.

At the same time, the separation of elderly people with significant mental infirmity from existing residential settings would probably benefit the non-demented elderly in care, since research indicates that increases in the proportion of confused residents in homes for the elderly tend to reduce levels of activity and communication amongst residents (Wilkin, Hughes and Evans, 1981). The stigma of 'psychogeriatric' ghettoes in local authority homes is, of course, a matter of due concern, but policies of segregation do not automatically produce degraded institutional care services. In any case, the present segregation of significant numbers of elderly mentally infirm people in psychogeriatric long-stay wards is already a feature of the current care system which adds the stigma of mental hospitalisation to that of the segregation that is an intrinsic feature of such hospital care.

Training Needs

Returning to the circle of care, need and responsibility, it is apparent that a model of family counselling, developed within a community psychogeriatric service, could provide help in both resolving interpersonal dynamics that may cloud the objective appraisal of need and responsibility, and in developing caregiving skills that could enhance the sense of positive coping and esteem arising from an increasing ability of carers to meet effectively these needs and responsibilities.

Such skills need to be developed during the training of prospective psychogeriatricians, clinical psychologists, social workers and nurses, and the community psychogeriatic day centre may be an ideal focus for developing such training experience. Here, statutory-service providers meet the informal primary caregivers, and inevitably have to work together to manage and share responsibility for the care of the dementing person.

The present organic orientation and the dispensing of services as if they were pills mitigate against a more psychologically sensitive approach to psychogeriatrics. A narrow focus on the dementing person as patient may foster such an impersonal approach to care, since it is difficult to develop any sense of a personal relationship between patient/client and physician/caseworker when the meeting takes place after the person has deteriorated. A shift of emphasis to the family context, and recognition of the other victims of dementia, can provide the setting conditions for an inevitably more personalised approach.

The day centre provides a meeting point between family care and statutory care when ownership of 'the bed' still remains in family hands, and as such leads to an increasing sharing of what problems exist. Need is thus likely to develop from a shared perspective by carer and staff, and caregiving or care-managing may thus be practised within this framework, a position difficult to sustain once the services 'own the bed', and thus manage the care system with the resulting staff-oriented perception of need.

Under these circumstances, day care, freed from responsibility to a psychiatric or geriatric hospital, can act as the base for psychogeriatric community care while maintaining control over residential places, in a way that it cannot under the present domination of the parent hospital. The existence of such a non-hospital base further permits a phased introduction to small-scale residential care, and a means of sustaining relationships between staff and family during this intermediate stage of partial institutionalisation. Day care will not then be seen as failing, if and when a dementing person enters full-time residential care. If staff are allowed to work in both residential and day care settings, they in turn can be agents of continuity in the care stystem, with an awareness of the history and dynamics of pre-existing family relationships within which the elderly patients' mental deterioration has taken place. Ideally too, staff would have been trained in both nursing and social-work skills, giving them a greater flexibility in their professional activities, and an equal appreciation of the physical and social dimensions of dementia. While it still seems desirable that such services be integrated by a consultant psychogeriatrician, it is probable that much day-to-day decision-making could be delegated to senior care workers/nurses with this type of background training.

Summary

A model has been proposed for developing a community psychogeriatric service which is family-oriented and which recognises the need for a care system that can encompass the decline of dementia from its initial identification to death. It is based upon the premise that dementia is fundamentally the erosion of self, whose management requires an increasingly supervisory and supportive agency to take responsibility for the dementing person's behaviour as their intending and adapting self fades. The difficulties and limitations of family carers that are evinced in this process are sufficiently stressful for the majority of carers to require some form of professional intervention, but one based upon developing a shared commitment to the supervisory and supportive aspects of caring at a rate which permits the principal carer to maintain their caring role as they have the desire and resources to do so.

The model system explicitly recognises that caregiving moves inevitably towards a 24-hour responsibility, which may only be realised in the less demanding environment of residential care. However, this does not in itself require a hospital model of care. The importance of maintaining continuity of professional interest is stressed from identification through to residential management and terminal care, and the value of providing staff with work settings which can encompass this shared-care system is underlined. Thus residential, day care and community workers should not have to be different people, occupying different professional roles. Those responsible for caregiving – in the form of supportive and supervisory behaviours – should not be removed from the opportunity of care-managing, and vice versa. Thus family members need to be involved in sustaining the system, both within day care and within residential settings, and need to be given the opportunity to determine and develop policy in both these settings.

Finally, it can be argued that the cost implications of running (as opposed to instituting) such a care system are not excessively greater than current costs expended on the dementing elderly who are identified by existing services. The benefits are primarily the recognition that a service can be created which provides a full appreciation of dementia, taking the place of the current fragmented system of care which currently denies the opportunity for continuity of care and offers instead a series of impersonal and uncoordinated 'things to be done'. Living with dementia is coming to terms with the irreversible loss of a human being. In many ways, professionals themselves shelter from that experience and thereby consign families and carers to the periphery of the community, isolated units for whom things are done by distant and differing agencies, with little sustained care and recognition of the problems involved.

When this system breaks down, an equally isolated switch is made to institutional care, given begrudgingly and sustaining the notion that relatives are being put away. The dearth of institutional beds in Britain has inevitably created a sense of their 'undesirability' and community care is offered as a more humane system, or indeed as the only caring system. Inevitably, guilt is created in relatives when this system breaks down, and the unacceptable has to be accepted. By making the care system more coherent and continuous, the transfer of responsibility can be made into a positive decision, one which minimises and cushions all the victims of dementia from perceiving such developments as failure, and allows the community to meet the loss of dementia with a positive and objective response and a more rational care system.

APPENDIX

Measures used in the Edinburgh studies are described in detail in this appendix, to indicate the means used to gather information on problems, strain and services as reported by the supporting relatives.

Problem Checklist

Each item is rated as either 'not present', 'occasionally occurring' or 'frequently/ continually occurring' – scored 0, 1 or 2. Those situations which occur at least occasionally are then rated as 'no problem', 'a small problem' or 'a great problem'.

1. Unable to dress without help
2. Demands attention
3. Unable to get in and out of a chair without help
4. Uses bad language
5. Unable to get in and out of bed without help
6. Disrupts personal and social life
7. Unable to wash without help
8. Physically aggressive
9. Needs help at mealtimes
10. Vulgar habits (e.g. spitting, table manners)
11. Incontinent – soiling
12. Creates personality clashes
13. Forgets things that have happened
14. Temper outbursts
15. Falling
16. Rude to visitors
17. Unable to manage stairs
18. Not safe if outside the house alone
19. Cannot be left alone for even one hour
20. Wanders about the house at night
21. Careless about own appearance
22. Unable to walk outside house
23. Unable to hold a sensible conversation
24. Noisy, shouting
25. Incontinent – wetting
26. Shows no concern for personal hygiene
27. Unsteady on feet
28. Always asking questions
29. Unable to take part in family conversations
30. Unable to read newspapers, magazines, etc.
31. Sits around doing nothing
32. Shows no interest in news about friends and relatives
33. Unable to watch and follow television (or radio)
34. Unable to occupy himself/herself doing useful things

Strain Scale

The items were derived from Machin's scale (1980): response points were altered from 5 to 3 and some items omitted. Responses to each item were: 'a great deal of the time', 'sometimes' and 'never'. Scoring for item 9 is reversed.

Dangers
1. Do you fear accidents or dangers concerning the elderly person (e.g. fire, gas, falling over, etc.)?

Embarrassment
2. Do you ever feel embarrassed by the elderly person in any way?

Sleep
3. Is your sleep ever interrupted by the elderly person?

Coping
4. How often do you feel it is difficult to cope with the situation you are in and in particular with the elderly person?

Depression
5. Do you ever get depressed about the situation?

Worry
6. How much do you worry about the elderly person?

Household Routine
7. Has your household routine been upset in caring for the elderly relative?

Frustration
8. Do you feel frustrated with your situation?

Enjoyment of Role
9. Do you get any pleasure from caring for the elderly person?

Holidays
10. Do the problems of caring prevent you from getting away on holiday?

Finance
11. Has your standard of living been affected in any way due to the necessity of caring for your elderly relative?

Health
12. Would you say that your health had suffered from looking after your relative?

Attention
13. Do you find the demand for companionship and attention from the elderly person gets too much for you?

Formal Services Received

An index of statutory support based upon the relatives' reports (NB: no external validation).

	Visits weekly or oftener (2)	Visits monthly or oftener (1)	No visits (0)
General practitioner			
District nurse			
Health visitor			
Social worker			
Home help			
Chiropodist			
Hairdresser			
Meals-on-wheels			

The 'score' is based upon the number of visiting services and their frequency – potential range from 0 to 16: actual range 0 to 10.

REFERENCES

Abrams, M. (1978) *Beyond Three Score and Ten*, Age Concern Publications, Mitcham, Surrey

Adolfsson, R., Kajsajuntti, G., Larsson, N., Myrstener, A., Nystrom, L., Oloffson, B.-O., Sandman, P.-O. and Winberg, J. (1980) 'Anhongas synpunkter pa amhandertagondet av aldersdementa', *Svenska Lakartidningen, 28/29*, 2519–21

Adolfsson, R., Gottfries, C.-G, Nystrom, L. and Winblad, B. (1981) 'Prevalence of dementia disorders in institutionalised Swedish old people', *Acta Psychiatrica Scandinavica, 63*, 225–44

Age Concern (1983) *Mental Health in Old Age: A Collection of Projects*, Age Concern Publications, Mitcham, Surrey

Allan, G. (1983) 'Informal networks of care: issues raised by Barclay', *British Journal of Social Work, 13*, 417–34

Aminoff, M. J., Marshall, J., Smith, E.M. and Wyke, M.A. (1975) 'Pattern of intellectual impairment in Huntington's chorea', *Psychological Medicine, 6*, 214–17

Archbold, P.G. (1981) 'Impact of parent caring on women', Paper presented at the XII International Congress of Gerontology, Hamburg, West Germany, July 1981

Ball, M.J. (1977) 'Neuronal loss, neurofibrillary tangles and granulovacuolar degeneration in the hippocampus with aging and dementia: a quantitiative study', *Acta Neuropathologia* (Berlin), *37*, 111–18

Ballinger, B.R., Cameron, L., Munro, A.N. and Scott, J.C. (1981) 'Inter-district comparison of geriatric psychiatry services', *Health Bulletin* (Edinburgh), *39*, 228–35

Ballinger, B.R., Reid, A.H. and Heather, B.B. (1982) Cluster analysis of symptoms in elderly demented patients', *British Journal of Psychiatry, 140*, 257–62

Barber, J.H. and Wallis, J.B. (1978) 'The benefits to an elderly population of continuing geriatric assessment', *Journal of the Royal College of General Practitioners, 28*, 428–33

Barber, J.H. and Wallis, J.B. (1982) 'The effects of a system of geriatric screening and assessment on general practice workload', *Health Bulletin* (Edinburgh), *40*, 125–32

Barclay, P.M. (1982) *Social Workers, their Role and Tasks*, Bedford Square Press for National Institute of Social Work, London

Barnes, R., Raskind, M., Scott, M. and Murphy, C. (1981) 'Problems of families caring for Alzheimer patients: use of a support group', *Journal of the American Geriatrics Society, 29*, 80–5

Barnes, R., Veith, R., Okinoto, J., Raskind, M. and Gumbrecht, G. (1982) 'Efficacy of antipsychotic medication in behaviorally disturbed dementia patients', *American Journal of Psychiatry, 139*, 1170–4

Bebbington, A.C. (1979) 'Changes in the provision of domiciliary social services to the community over fourteen years', *Social Policy and Administration, 13*, 111–23

Bergmann, K., Foster, E.M., Justice, A.W. and Mathews, V. (1978) 'Management of the elderly demented patient in the community', *British Journal of Psychiatry, 132*, 441–9

Bergmann, K., Kay, B.W.K., Foster, E.M., McKechnie, A.A. and Roth, M. (1971) 'A follow-up study of randomly selected community residents to assess the effects of chronic brain syndrome and cerebrovascular disease', *Excerpta Medica Inter-*

125

national Congress Series, no. 274, Psychiatry (pt II), 856–65

Birkett, D.P. (1972) 'The psychiatric differentiation of senility and arteriosclerosis', *British Journal of Psychiatry, 120*, 321–5

Blenkner, M., Bloom, M., Wesser, E. and Nielson, M. (1971) 'A research and demonstration project of protective services', *Social Casework, 52*, 483–99

Blumenthal, M.D. (1979) 'Psychosocial factors in reversible and irreversible brain failure', *Journal of Clinical and Experimental Gerontology, 1*, 39–55

Bond, J. and Carstairs, V. (1982) *Services for the Elderly*, Scottish Health Services Studies, no. 42, SHHD, Edinburgh

Bradshaw, J.R., Thomson, J.L.G. and Campbell, M.J. (1983) 'Computerised tomography in the investigation of dementia', *British Medical Journal, 286*, 277–80

Brocklehurst J.C. (1970) *The Geriatric Day Hospital*, King Edward's Hospital Fund for London, London

Brocklehurst, J.C. (1973) 'Geriatric services and the day hospital', in J.C. Brocklehurst (ed.), *Textbook of Geriatric Medicine and Gerontology*, Churchill Livingstone, Edinburgh, 673–91

Brocklehurst, J.C. and Tucker, J.S. (1980) *Progress in Geriatric Day Care*, King Edward's Hospital Fund for London, London

Brodie, H.M. (1978) 'Cell counts in cerebral cortex and brainstem in Alzheimer's disease, senile dementia and related disorders', in R. Katzman, R.D. Terry, and K.L. Brick (eds.), *Alzheimer's Disease, Senile Dementia and Related Disorders*, Raven Press, New York

Burnside, I.M. (1980) 'Symptomatic behaviors in the elderly', in J.E. Birren and R.B. Sloane (eds.), *Handbook of Mental Health and Aging*, Prentice-Hall, Englewood Cliffs, NJ, 719–44

Campbell, A.J., McGosh, L.M., Reinker, J. and Allan, B.C. (1983) 'Dementia in old age and the need for services', *Age and Ageing, 12*, 11–16

Challis, D.J. and Davies, B. (1980) 'A new approach to community care of the elderly', *British Journal of Social Work, 10*, 1–18

Charlesworth, A. and Wilkin, D. (1982) *Dependency among old people in geriatric wards, psychogeriatric wards and residential homes, 1977–1981*, Research Report no. 6, University Hospital of South Manchester, Psychogeriatric Unit —Research Section

Christie, A.B. (1982) 'Changing patterns of mental illness in the elderly', *British Journal of Psychiatry, 140*, 154–9

Clark, J. (1981) *What do Health Visitors Do?* Royal College of Nursing, London

Clarke, M.G., Williams, A.J. and Jones, P.A. (1981) 'A psychogeriatric survey of old people's homes', *British Medical Journal, 283*, 1307–9

Constantinidis, J. (1978) 'Is Alzheimer's disease a major form of senile dementia? Clinical, anatomical and genetic data', in R. Katzman, R.D. Terry and K.C. Brick (eds.), *Alzheimer's Disease, Senile Dementia and Related Disorders*, Raven Press, New York

Crosbie, D. (1983) 'A role for anyone? A description of social work with the elderly in two area offices', *British Journal of Social Work, 13*, 123–48

DHSS (1972) 'Services for mental illness related to old age', circular HM(72)71

DHSS (1981) *Growing Older*, HMSO, London

Diesfeldt, H.F. (1978) 'The distinction between long-term and short-term memory in senile dementia: an analysis of free recall and delayed recognition', *Neuropsychologia, 16*, 115–19

Eagles, J.M. (1983) 'Factors affecting the admission and discharge, placements of demented patients in a psychogeriatric assessment unit', unpublished MPhil thesis, University of Edinburgh

Edwards, C., Sinclair, I. and Gorbach, P. (1980) 'Day centres for the elderly: variations in type, provision and users' response', *British Journal of Social Work*,

10, 419–30

Farndale, J. (1961) *The Day Hospital Movement in Great Britain*, Pergamon Press, New York

Fengler, A.P. and Goodrich, N. (1979) 'Wives of elderly disabled men: the hidden patients', *Gerontologist*, *19*, 175–83

Fennell, G., Emerson, A.R., Sidell, M. and Hague, A. (1981) *Day Centres for the Elderly in East Anglia*, Centre for East Anglian Studies, Norwich

Foster, E.M., Kay, D.W.K. and Bergmann, K. (1976) 'The characteristics of old people receiving and needing domiciliary services: the relevance of psychiatric diagnosis', *Age and Ageing*, *5*, 245–51

Foulds, G.A. (1976) *The Hierarchical Nature of Personal Illness*, Academic Press, London

Gaspar, D. (1980) 'Hollymoor Hospital dementia service', *The Lancet*, *i*, 1402–5

General Household Survey, 1980 and 1981, Office of Population Censuses and Surveys, Social Services Division, HMSO, London, 1982 and 1983

Gilhooley, M.L.M. (1980) 'The social dimensions of senile dementia', Paper presented at the British Psychological Society Annual Conference, Aberdeen, March 1980

Gilhooley, M.L.M. (1981) 'The social dimensions of senile dementia', Paper presented at the XII International Congress of Gerontology, Hamburg, West Germany, July 1981

Gilhooley, M.L.M. (1984a) 'The impact of caregiving on caregivers: factors associated with the psychological well-being of people supporting a dementing relative in the community', *British Journal of Medical Psychology* (in press)

Gilhooley, M.L.M. (1984b) 'Senile dementia: factors associated with supporters' willingness to consider institutionalisation', *Social Science and Medicine* (in press)

Gilleard, C.J. (1978) 'An investigation into the nature of behavioural change in the dementias of old age', PhD thesis, University of Leeds

Gilleard, C.J. (1981) 'Incontinence in the hospitalised elderly', *Health Bulletin* (Edinburgh), *39*, 58–61

Gilleard, C.J. (1983) 'Evaluation of psychogeriatric daycare', Paper presented at the 1st International Conference on Systems Science in Health Care, Canada, July

Gilleard, C.J. (1984) 'Assessment of behavioural impairment in the elderly', in: I.G. Hanley and J. Hodge (eds.), *Psychology Applied to the Care of the Elderly*, Croom Helm, London

Gilleard, C.J. and Pattie, A.H. (1978) 'The effect of location on the elderly mentally infirm', *Age and Ageing*, *7*, 1–6

Gilleard, C.J. and Watt, G. (1982) 'The impact of psychogeriatric day-care on the primary supporter of the elderly mentally infirm', in R. Taylor and A. Gilmore (eds.), *Current Trends in British Gerontology*, Gower Publishing, Aldershot, 139–47

Gilleard, C.J., Boyd, W.D. and Watt, G. (1982) 'Problems in caring for the elderly mentally infirm at home', *Archives of Gerontology and Geriatrics*, *1*, 151–8

Gillespie, J.V. (1980) 'Night nursing service in West Fife', *Health Bulletin*, *38*, 187–93

Gillis, L.S., Elk, R., Trinchard, L., LeFevre, K., Zabow, A., Jaffe, H. and Van Schalkwyk, D. (1982) 'The admission of the elderly to places of care: a sociopsychiatric community study', *Psychological Medicine*, *12*, 159–68

Goldberg, D.P. (1978) *Manual for the General Health Questionnaire*, NFER–Nelson, Windsor

Grad, J. d'Alarcon and Sainsbury, P. (1965) 'An evaluation of the effects of caring for the aged at home', in *Psychiatric Disorders in the Aged*, WPA Symposium, Geigy, Manchester

Greene, J.G. and Timbury, G.C. (1979) 'A geriatric psychiatry day hospital service: a five year review', *Age and Ageing, 8,* 49–53

Greene, J.G., Smith, R., Gardiner, M. and Timbury, G.C. (1982) 'Measuring behavioural disturbance of elderly demented patients in the community and its effects on relatives: a factor analytic study', *Age and Ageing, 11,* 121–6

Greene, J.G., Timbury, G.C., Smith, R. and Gardiner, M. (1983) 'Reality orientation with elderly patients in the community: an empirical evaluation', *Age and Ageing, 12,* 38–43

Gruer, R. (1975) *Needs of the Elderly in the Scottish Borders,* Scottish Health Services Studies, no. 33, SHHD, Edinburgh

Grundy, E. and Arie, T. (1982) 'Falling rate of provision of residential care for the elderly', *British Medical Journal, 284,* 779–802

Guntrip, H. (1971) *Psychoanalytic Theory, Therapy and the Self,* Hogarth Press, London

Gurland, B. (1980) 'The assessment of the mental health status of older adults', in J.E. Birren and R.B. Sloane (eds.), *Handbook of Mental Health and Aging,* Prentice-Hall, Englewood Cliffs, NJ, 671–700

Gustafson, L. and Hagberg, B. (1975) 'Emotional behaviour, personality changes and cognitive reduction in presenile dementia: related to regional cerebral blood flow', *Acta Psychiatrica Scandinavica,* Supplement 257

Gustafson, L. and Nilsson, L. (1982) 'Differential diagnosis of presenile dementia on clinical grounds', *Acta Psychiatrica Scandinavica, 65,* 194–209

Hachinski, V.C., Iliff, L.P., Zilhka, E., du Boulay, G.H., McAllister, V.L., Marshall, J., Ross-Russell, R.W. and Syrian, L. (1975) 'Cerebral blood flow in dementia', *Archives of Neurology, 32,* 632–7

Hagberg, B. and Ingvar, D.H. (1976) 'Cognitive reductions in presenile dementia related to regional abnormalities of the cerebral blood flow' *British Journal of Psychiatry, 127,* 209–21

Hanley, T. (1974) 'Neuronal fallout in the ageing brain: a critical review of the quantitative data', *Age and Ageing, 3,* 133–51

Harrison, M.J.G., Thomas, D.J., du Boulay, G.H. and Marshall, J. (1979) 'Multi-infarct dementia', *Journal of Neurological Science, 40,* 97–103

Hasegawa, K. and Homma, A. (1981) 'A gerontopsychiatric five years follow-up study on age-related dementia', Paper presented at the XII International Congress of Gerontology, Hamburg, West Germany, July 1981

Helgason, T. (1977) 'Psychiatric services and mental illness in Iceland', *Acta Psychiatrica Scandinavica,* Supplement 268

Hemsi, L. (1982) 'Psychogeriatric care in the community', in R. Levy and F. Post (eds.), *The Psychiatry of Late Life,* Blackwell Scientific Publications, London, 252–87

Heston, L.L., Mastri, A.R., Anderson, E. and White, J. (1981) 'Dementia of the Alzheimer type: clinical genetics, natural history and associated conditions', *Archives of General Psychiatry, 38,* 1085–90

Hilgard, E., Atkinson, R.C. and Atkinson, R.L. (1975) *Introduction to Psychology,* 6th edn, Harcourt Brace Jovanovich, New York

Hirschfeld, M.J. (1981) 'Families living and coping with the cognitively impaired', in L. Archer Copp (ed.), *Recent Advances in Nursing, 2, Care of the Ageing,* Churchill Livingstone, Edinburgh, 159–67

Horowitz, A. (1981) 'Sons and daughters as caregivers to older parents: differences in role performance and consequences', Paper presented at the 34th Annual Scientific Meeting of the Gerontological Society of America, Toronto, Canada, November 1981

Horowitz, A. (1982) 'The impact of caregiving on children of the frail elderly', Paper presented at the Annual Meeting of the American Orthopsychiatric Association,

San Francisco, USA, March 1982

Horowitz, A. and Shindelman, L.W. (1981) 'Reciprocity and affection: past influences on current caregiving', Paper presented at the 34th Annual Scientific Meeting of the Gerontological Society of America, Toronto, Canada, November 1981

Ikegami, N. (1982) 'Institutionalized and the non-institutionalized elderly', *Social Science and Medicine, 16*, 2001–8

Inglis, J. (1958) 'Learning retention and conceptual usage in elderly patients with memory disorder', *Journal of Abnormal and Social Psychology, 59*, 210–15

Isaacs, B. (1971) 'Geriatric patients: do their families care?' *British Medical Journal, 4*, 282–5

Isaacs, B., Livingston, M. and Neville, Y. (1972) *Survival of the Unfittest: a study of geriatric patients in the East End of Glasgow*, Routledge and Kegan Paul, London

Jerrome, D. (1981) 'The significance of friendship for women in later life', *Ageing and Society, 1*, 175–98

Johnson, C.L. (1983) 'Dyadic family relations and social support', *Gerontologist, 23*, 377–83

Johnson, C.L. and Catalona, D.J. (1982) 'A longitudinal study of family supports to impaired elderly', Paper presented at the 35th Annual Scientific Meeting of the Gerontological Society of America, Boston, USA, November 1982

Jones, I.G. and Munbodh, R. (1982) 'An evaluation of a day hospital for the demented elderly', *Health Bulletin* (Edinburgh), *40*, 10–15

Jonsson, O.-C., Waldton, S. and Malhammer, G. (1973) 'The psychiatric symptomatology in senile dementia assessed by means of an interview', *Acta Psychiatrica Scandinavica, 48*, 103–21

Kahn, R.L. and Tobin, S.S. (1981) 'Community treatment for aged persons with altered brain function', in N.E. Miller and G.D. Cohen (eds.), *Clinical Aspects of Alzheimer's Disease and Senile Dementia*, Raven Press, New York, 253–76

Kahn, R.L., Goldfarb, A.L., Pollack, M. and Gerber, I.E. (1960) 'Brief objective measures for the determination of mental status in the aged', *American Journal of Psychiatry, 117*, 326–8

Kasniack, A.W., Fox, J., Gandell, D.L., Garron, D.C., Huckman, M.S. and Ramsey, R.G. (1978) 'Predictors of mortality in presenile and senile dementia', *Annals of Neurology, 3*, 246–52

Kay, D.W.K. and Bergmann, K. (1980) 'Epidemiology of mental disorders amongst the aged in the community', in J.E. Birren and R.B. Sloane (eds.), *Handbook of Mental Health and Aging*, Prentice-Hall, Englewood Cliffs, NJ, 34–56

Kay, D.W.K., Beamish, P. and Roth, M. (1964) 'Old age mental disorders in Newcastle upon Tyne part I. A study of prevalence', *British Journal of Psychiatry, 110*, 146–58

Kay, D.W.K., Bergmann, K., Foster, E.M., McKechnie, A.A. and Roth, M. (1970) 'Mental illness and hospital usage in the elderly: a random sample followed up', *Comprehensive Psychiatry, 11*, 26–35

Kellett, J.M., Copeland, J.R.M. and Kelleher, M.J. (1975) 'Information leading to accurate diagnosis in the elderly', *British Journal of Psychiatry, 126*, 423–30

Klusmann, D., Bruder, J., Lauter, H. and Luders, I. (1981) 'Beziehungen zwischen Patienten und ihren Familienangehorigen bei chronischen Erkrankungen des hoheren Lebensalters', Teilprojekt A16, Sonderforschungsbereich, 115 der Deutschen Forschungsgemeinschaft, Hamburg

Koopman-Boyden, P.G. and Wells, L.F. (1979) 'The problems arising from supporting the elderly at home', *New Zealand Medical Journal, 89*, 265–8

Kral, V.A. (1962) 'Senescent forgetfulness: benign and malignant', *Canadian Medical Association Journal, 86*, 257–60

Larsson, T., Sjogren, T. and Jacobson, G. (1963) 'Senile dementia: a clinical, socio-medical and genetic study', *Acta Psychiatrica Scandinavica*, Supplement 167, 1–259

LaRue, A. and Jarvik, L.F. (1980) 'Reflections of biological changes in the psychological performance of the aged', *Age, 3*, 29–32

Latto, S.M. (1981) 'Managing the care system', in F. Glendenning (ed.), *Care in the Community: Recent Research and Current Projects*, Beth Johnson Foundation Publications, Hartshill, 61–71

Lauter, H. and Meyer, J.E. (1968) 'Clinical and nosological concepts of senile dementia', in C. Muller and L. Ciompi (eds.), *Senile Dementia: Clinical and Therapeutic Aspects*, Hans Huber, Berne

Lawton, M.P. and Nahemow, L. (1973) 'Ecology and the aging process', in C. Eisdorfer and M.P. Lawton (eds.), *The Psychology of Adult Development and Aging*, American Psychological Association, Washington

Lazarus, R.S. and DeLongis, A. (1982) 'Psychological stress and coping in aging', *American Psychologist, 38*, 245–54

Lieberman, M.A. (1975) 'Adaptive processes in late life', in N. Datan and L. Ginsborg (eds.), *Life Span Developmental Psychology: Normative Life Crises*, Academic Press, New York

Liston, E.J. (1977) 'Occult presenile dementia', *Journal of Nervous and Mental Disease, 164*, 263–7

Luker, K.A. (1981) 'The role of the health visitor', in J. Kinnaird, J. Brotherston and J. Williamson (eds.), *The Provision of Care for the Elderly*, Churchill Livingstone, Edinburgh

Luria, A.R. (1973) *The Working Brain*, Penguin, Harmondsworth

MacDonald, A.J.D., Mann, A.H., Jenkins, R., Richard, L., Godlove, C. and Rodwell, G. (1982) 'An attempt to determine the impact of four types of care upon the elderly', *Psychological Medicine, 12*, 193–200

McDonald, C. (1969) 'Clinical heterogeneity in senile dementia' *British Journal of Psychiatry, 115*, 267–71

McLaren, S.M., McPherson, F.M., Sinclair, F. and Ballinger, B.R. (1981) 'Prevalence and severity of incontinence among hospitalised female psychogeriatric patients', *Health Bulletin* (Edinburgh) *39*, 157–61

Macmillan, D. (1960) 'Preventive geriatrics: opportunities of a community mental health service', *The Lancet, ii*, 1439–41

Macmillan, D. (1967) 'Problems of a geriatric mental health service', *British Journal of Psychiatry, 113*, 175–81

Mace, N. and Robins, P. (1981) *The 36-Hour Day*, Johns Hopkins University Press, Baltimore

Machin, E. (1980) 'A survey of the behaviour of the elderly and their supporters at home', unpublished MSc thesis, University of Birmingham

Maeda, D. (1978) 'Ageing in eastern society', in D. Hobman (ed.), *The Social Challenge of Ageing*, Croom Helm, London, 45–72

Makizano, K. (1978) 'Division of household: an evidence of the weakening social norm of family support and care of aged parents', Paper presented at the XI International Congress of Gerontology, Tokyo, Japan, July 1978

Masterton, G.K., Holloway, E.M. and Timbury, G.C. (1979) 'The prevalence of organic cerebral impairment and behavioural problems within local authority homes for the elderly', *Age and Ageing, 8*, 226–30

Meacher, M. (1972) *Taken for a Ride: Special Residential Homes for Confused Old People*, Longmans, London

Mead, G.M. and Castleden, C.M. (1982) 'Confusion and hypnotics and dementia patients', *Journal of the Royal College of General Practitioners, 32*, 763–5

Miller, E. (1971) 'On the nature of the memory disorder in presenile dementia', *Neuropsychologia, 9*, 75–81

Miller, E. (1975) 'Impaired recall and memory disturbance in presenile dementia', *British Journal of Social and Clinical Psychology, 14*, 73–9

Miller, E. (1977) *Abnormal Ageing: the Psychology of Senile and Presenile Dementia*, Wiley, Chichester

Morris, R., Wheatley, J. and Britton, P.G. (1983) 'Retrieval from long-term memory in senile dementia: cued recall revisited', *British Journal of Clinical Psychology, 22*, 141–2

Muller, C. (1967) *Alterpsychiatrie*, Georg Thieme Verlag, Stuttgart

Naguib, M. and Levy, R. (1982) 'Prediction of outcome in senile dementia: a computed tomography study', *British Journal of Psychiatry, 140*, 263–7

Nielson, J., Homma, A. and Biorn-Henrikson, T. (1977) 'Follow-up 15 years after a geronto-psychiatric prevalence study: conditions concerning death, cause of death, and life expectancy in relation to psychiatric diagnosis', *Journal of Gerontology, 32*, 554–61

OPCS (1983) *Social Trends, 12*, HMSO, London, 14

Opit, L.J. (1977) 'Domiciliary care for the elderly sick: economy or neglect?' *British Medical Journal, 1*, 30–3

Pearlin, L.I. and Schooler, C. (1978) 'The structure of coping', *Journal of Health and Social Behaviour, 19*, 2–21

Perez, F.I., Rivera, V.M., Meyer, J.S., Gay, J.R.A., Taylor, R.L. and Mathew, N.T. (1975) 'Analysis of intellectual and cognitive performance in patients with multi-infarct dementia, vertebro-basilar insufficiency with dementia, and Alzheimer's disease', *Journal of Neurology, Neurosurgery and Psychiatary, 38*, 533–40

Reifler, B.V., Cox, G.B. and Hanley, R.S. (1981) 'Problems of the mentally ill elderly as perceived by patients, family and clinicians', *Gerontologist, 21*, 165–70

Reifler, B.V., Larson, E. and Hanley, R.S. (1982) 'Co-existence of cognitive impairment and depression in geriatric outpatients', *American Journal of Psychiatry, 139*, 623–6

Reisberg, B., Ferris, S.H., De Leon, M.J. and Crook, T. (1982) 'The global deterioration scale for assessment of primary degenerative dementia', *American Journal of Psychiatry, 139*, 1136–9

Robinson, B.C. (1983) 'Validation of a caregiver strain index', *Journal of Gerontology, 38*, 344–8

Ross, D.N. (1976) 'Geriatric day hospitals: counting the cost compared with other methods of support', *Age and Ageing, 5*, 171–5

Ross, H.E. and Kedward, H.B. (1977) 'Psychogeriatric hospital admissions from the community and institutions', *Journal of Gerontology, 32*, 420–7

Rossor, M.N. (1982) 'Dementia', *The Lancet, ii*, 1200–4

Roth, M. (1955) 'The natural history of mental disorder in old age', *Journal of Mental Science, 101*, 281–301

Sainsbury, P., Costain, W.R. and Grad, J. d'Alarcon (1965) 'The effects of a community service on the referral and admission rates of elderly psychiatric patients', in *Psychiatric Disorders of the Aged*, WPA Symposium, Geigy, Manchester, 23–37

Sanford, J.R.A. (1975) 'Tolerance of debility in elderly dependants by supporters at home: its significance for hospital practice', *British Medical Journal, 3*, 471–5

Schneck, M.K., Reisberg, B. and Ferris, S.H. (1982) 'An overview of current concepts of Alzheimer's disease', *American Journal of Psychiatry, 139*, 165–73

Scottish Abstract of Statistics: 1973–1981. Scottish Office, HMSO, Edinburgh

Seligman, M.E.P. (1975) *Helplessness*, W.H. Freeman, San Francisco

Semple, S.A., Smith, C.M. and Swash, M. (1982) 'The Alzheimer disease syndrome', in S. Corkin, K.L. Davis, J.H. Growdon, E. Usdin and R.J. Wurtman (eds.), *Alzheimer's Disease: A Report of Progress and Research*, Raven Press,

New York, 93–108

Shah, K.V., Banks, G.P. and Merskey, H. (1969) 'Survival in atherosclerotic and senile dementia', *British Journal of Psychiatry, 115*, 1283–6

Sheldon, J.H. (1948) *The Social Medicine of Old Age*, Oxford University Press, London

SHHD (1970) *Services for the Elderly with Mental Disorder*, HMSO, Edinburgh

Smith, G. (1980) *Social Need*, Routledge and Kegan Paul, London

Smith, G. (1982) 'Some problems in the evaluation of a new psychogeriatric day hospital', in R. Taylor and A. Gilmore (eds.), *Current Trends in British Gerontology*, Gower Publishing, Aldershot, 204–16

Smith, J.S. and Kiloh, L.G. (1981) 'The investigation of dementia; results in 200 consecutive admissions', *The Lancet, ii*, 824–7

Symonds, R.L. (1981) 'Dementia as an experience', *Nursing Times*, 30 September, 1708–10

Thom, W.T. (1981) 'Housing Policies', in J. Kinnaird, J. Brotherston and J. Williamson (eds.), *The Provision of Care for the Elderly*, Churchill Livingstone, Edinburgh, 38–43

Thompson, E.G. and Eastwood, M.R. (1981) 'Survivorship and senile dementia', *Age and Ageing, 10*, 29–32

Tibbett, J.E. and Tombs, J. (1981) *Day Services for the Elderly and Elderly with Mental Disability in Scotland*, Central Research Unit, Scottish Office, HMSO, Edinburgh

Tulloch, A.J. and Moore, V. (1979) 'A randomized controlled trial of geriatric screening and surveillance in general practice', *Journal of the Royal College of General Practitioners, 29*, 730–3

Turner, R.J. and Sternberg, M.P. (1978) 'Psychosocial factors in elderly patients admitted to a psychiatric hospital', *Age and Ageing, 7*, 171–7

Vetter, N.J., Jones, D.A. and Victor, C.R. (1981), 'Variations in care for the elderly in Wales, *Journal of Epidemiology and Community Health, 35*, 128–32

Victoratos, G.C., Lenman, J.A.R. and Herzberg, L. (1977) 'Neurological investigation of dementia', *British Journal of Psychiatry, 130*, 131–3

Watt, G.M. (1982) 'A family-oriented approach to community care for the elderly mentally infirm', *Nursing Times, 78* (37), 1545–8

Wattis, J., Wattis, L. and Arie, T. (1981) 'Psychogeriatrics: a national survey of a new branch of psychiatry', *British Medical Journal, 282*, 1529–33

Weingartner, H., Kaye, W., Smallberg, S.A., Ebert, M.H., Gillin, J.C. and Sitaram, N. (1981) 'Memory failures in progressive idiopathic dementia', *Journal of Abnormal Psychology, 90*, 187–96

Wells, C.E. (1978) 'Chronic brain disease: an overview', *American Journal of Psychiatry, 135*, 1–12

Wells, C.E. (1982) 'Refinements in the diagnosis of dementia', *American Journal of Psychiatry, 139*, 621–2

Wertheimer, J. (1974) 'La démence senile et son évolution', *Revue Medicale Suisse Romande, 94*, 545–54

Whitehead, J.A. (1974) 'Community and hospital services in Brighton', *Nursing Times, 70*, 1340

Wilkin, D., Hughes, B. and Evans, G. (1981) 'Integration of confused and lucid elderly people in institutional care: effects on levels of activity and communication', Paper presented at the XII International Congress of Gerontology, Hamburg, July 1981

Williamson, J. (1981) 'Screening, surveillance and case-finding', in T. Arie (ed.), *Health Care of the Elderly: Essays on Old Age Medicine, Psychiatry and Services*, Croom Helm, London

Williamson, J., Stokoe, I.H., Gray, S., Fisher, M., Smith, A., McGhee, A. and Stephenson, E. (1964) 'Old people at home: their unreported needs', *The*

Lancet, i, 1117–20

Zarit, J.M. (1982) 'Family roles, social supports and their relation to caregivers' burden', Paper presented at the meeting of the Western Psychological Association, Sacramento, USA, July 1982

Zarit, J.M., Gatz, M. and Zarit, S.H. (1981) 'Family relationships and burden in long-term care', Paper presented at the 34th Annual Scientific Meeting of the Gerontological Society of America, Toronto, Canada, November 1981

Zarit, S.H., Reever, K.E. and Bach-Peterson, J. (1980) 'Relatives of the impaired elderly: correlates of feelings of burden', *Gerontologist, 20,* 649–55

INDEX